Strategies
for
Needs Assessment
in Prevention

The *Prevention in Human Services* series:

Strategies
for
Needs Assessment
in Prevention

Edited by
Alex Zautra
Kenneth Bachrach
Robert Hess

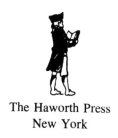

The Haworth Press
New York

Strategies for Needs Assessment in Prevention has also been published as *Prevention in Human Services,* Volume 2, Number 4, Summer 1983.

The Haworth Press, Inc., 28 East 22 Street, New York, NY 10010

Library of Congress Cataloging in Publication Data
Main entry under title:

Strategies for needs assessment in prevention.

"Strategies for needs assessment in prevention has also been published as Prevention in human services, volume 2, number 4, summer 1983"—P.
Includes bibliographies.
1. Mental health planning. 2. Community mental health services—Planning. 3. Social service—Planning.
I. Zautra, Alex. II. Bachrach, Kenneth. III. Hess, Robert, 1948-
RA790.5.S77 1983   362.2'0422   83-10861
ISBN 0-86656-187-0

Strategies for Needs Assessment in Prevention

Prevention in Human Services
Volume 2, Number 4

CONTENTS

Strategies
for
Needs Assessment
in Prevention

INTRODUCTION

The Role of Needs Assessment in Prevention

There are few in the field of prevention who have not had to puzzle over the question, "How do you solve a problem before it occurs?" The answer of course is that you cannot, at least not directly. The focus of prevention is on antecedent conditions that are thought to contribute to increased risk, and not on the problem itself. Individual vulnerabilities, chronic environmental strains and specific stressors, that some groups have and others do not, are targets for prevention activities. The rationale behind these prevention activities is that through interventions that alter antecedent conditions, problems are less likely to develop or are at least diminished in magnitude when they occur.

This approach is well known to prevention professionals. The empirical basis for selection of risk factors with which to work is much less secure, however. Antecedents are often chosen based on intuitively appealing but untested hypotheses or from plausible evidence gained from clinical casework rather than from studies of adequate sample size. There has been little quantitative data available to use in planning prevention programs.

Needs assessment investigations can fill this information gap by providing agencies with concrete data which test hypothesized relationships and uncover new ones. The process of conducting a needs assessment forces the prevention specialist to conceptualize the problem with greater clarity and supports the development of a theoretical framework to guide and test prevention activities.

In needs assessment, the question that plagues researchers is not very different from the one puzzling prevention workers, "How do you identify the problem before it occurs?" Armed with analytic tools and measurement instruments, the needs assessor searches first for factors associated with the problem. Next, the needs assessor employs theoretical, logical and statistical means to sift out the antecedents from the consequences of the problem. The goals are clear: to identify the conditions which precede and perhaps cause the problems which are to be prevented.

Background

The roots of needs assessment, particularly mental health needs assessment, are in epidemiology. As the name implies, epidemiology began as the study of epidemics; the discipline includes investigations of the distribution and determinants of states of health and disorder in the population. By definition this work is preventative. In the health field, factors associated with infection and the spread of disease are identified as well as the characteristics of particularly susceptible people. The hope is to reduce the number of new cases of the disorder by isolating people from suspected causes.

Full understanding of the etiology of the disorder is not necessary to identify antecedents, a point often made by way of analogy in support of mental health prevention activities. In a classic example, Snow in 1855 investigated the virulent epidemic of cholera in London which claimed 500 lives in less than 10 days (Roueche, 1958; Snow, 1855). He noted that most deaths occurred in a specific geographic area of London, in the neighborhood of Broad Street. Then, through interviews, he identified a common factor: the deceased had all used the Broad Street pump to obtain their drinking water. By closing the well Snow was able to immediately prevent new cases of cholera. This was 28 years before Koch's isolation of the cholera bacillus. There are many contemporary examples as well. The association between smoking and cancer is well known, for instance, even though the explicit biochemical processes linking them have not been fully identified.

There was early enthusiasm that the same type of epidemiological paradigm could be applied to problems without physiological manifestations. Investigators from the Chicago school of urban sociology examined spatial distributions of mental disorder (e.g., Faris & Dunham, 1939). They found geographically identifiable zones in the city that were associated with, and initially thought to cause, cases of mental disorder. In the same vein, Shevsky and Bell (1955) developed typologies of neighborhoods based on social area analyses of the economic, family and ethnic status of people living there.

There are several textbook examples of epidemiological investigations of mental disorder that were conducted in the 1950s and 1960s (e.g., Leighton, Harding, Macklin, MacMillan, & Leighton, 1963; Strole, Langner, Michael, Opler, & Rennie, 1962). Community samples were drawn and people were interviewed in their homes in attempts to measure the true prevalence of mental disorder in the general population.

Despite some weaknesses, these early studies were important in three respects. First, they showed that psychological distress was widespread and severe, even among those not receiving treatment. Second, the studies indicated that social factors such as income and education were associated with rates of mental disorder. Third, they found that those with the fewest social resources not only were most likely to be ill, but also least likely to find help for their problems. Mental health became a social problem.

These findings fit well with the progressive social philosophy of the time, encouraging significant developments in funding of community mental health programs. Programs were mandated to serve the needs of a geographically targeted area, often one that was poor and had few of its own resources.

The funding for establishing these centers, and the expansion of services within existing centers, relied on the demonstration of unmet need: that a significant proportion of the population in a center's catchment area was suffering from a mental disorder but was unable to obtain help from existing services. Under these auspices, needs assessment research was launched for the purposes of understanding and/or documenting a community's unmet needs. The use of social area analyses and advances in psychiatric epidemiology (Warheit, Bell, & Schwab, 1974) added methodological rigor to these investigations.

Much of this needs assessment work was not oriented toward the identification of antecedents of psychological problems but to the three *w*'s: *w*ho had *w*hat problems and *w*here did they live? These data were then used primarily to plan for the delivery of direct treatment services. Nevertheless, the identification of high risk population groups was and continues to be helpful to prevention planners, and information on the geographic distribution of problems aids in decisions on where to target programs. Examples of these types of needs assessment are contained in this volume.

Tighter fiscal resources have led to even more research activities to document unmet need, but perhaps less explicit attention to understanding the social problems of the community. In 1981, at the third national conference on needs assessment in Louisville, the word spread from conference participants working at NIMH that the new Republican administration was no longer funding "social" research on mental health. What this meant exactly is still unclear, but there was no doubt about the underlying message. Mental disorder was being unofficially declared no longer a social problem. The ramifications of this have yet to be fully realized.

These changes do nothing to diminish the usefulness of needs assessment, as Warheit and his colleagues point out in their contribution to this issue. The need for properly conducted and valid assessment of population needs is as important as ever. The purposes are different; before, these assessments were done to understand and promote expansion of services. Now these assessments are used to determine which existing services should be maintained and to defend innovative approaches in prevention because they are less costly than direct treatment.

Approaches to Identifying Needs

Four of the seven papers in this collection provide ways of defining and measuring psychological needs that hold much promise for prevention. The most straightforward approach is to define mental health needs based on whether or not a person displays signs of psychological distress or impairment that is comparable to the distress and impaired functioning of those who typically receive professional care. This definition is congruent with epidemiological models, and some of the papers in this volume are derivates of this basic strategy. In the lead article, Warheit, Vega and Buhl-Auth present one of the most thoroughly researched examples of this type. The authors synthesize some of the ground breaking research in the application of psychiatric epidemiology to needs assessment conducted by themselves and their colleagues. Based on an analysis of over 12,000 interviews with respondents from many different walks of life, they present a reliable method for identifying psycho-pathology and differentiating among its many forms. With a minimum of assumptions about human behavior, their approach succeeds as a methodology aimed at identifying who in the community is most likely to need what kind of help.

Evidence of distress in people is not the only indication of need and certainly not the earliest sign that something is wrong. A second major strategy to be considered is to identify conditions of life that either trouble people when present or disturb them when absent. Zautra and Sandler develop this view. They propose that a person's transactions with their environment should be used to plan preventative interventions. They present two life event models to guide needs assessments, one of which defines steps toward positive psychological growth. It accompanies the more familiar model depicting the process of adjustment to stressful life events.

The importance of social needs is being increasingly recognized by professionals and the lay public alike. There has been a growth in self-help groups in recent years and many prevention programs emphasize, in one form or another, the need for social support. Barrera and Balls review the research on this set of needs and present an example of social support research which should serve as a model for future prevention-oriented needs assessment. They identify a high risk group (pregnant teenagers), use multiple measures of social support to thoroughly assess need, and employ a prospective pre-post design to evaluate the predictive power of their measures. Their findings yield specific recommendations for how prevention programs could profitably intervene in the pregnancy.

The three papers described thus far use needs assessment as a research activity. In the next article, Martí-Costa and Serrano-García show how needs assessment has political purposes that depend on the values of the investigator. They propose an ordering of assessment methods dependent upon the degree to which information is used to strengthen existing institutions or encourage social change. From their perspective, central needs of individuals are to have control over their own lives and participation in the regulation of their own social institutions. To address these needs they employ techniques of needs assessment as tools for community development. Their approach provides a provocative view of how needs assessment can be applied to groups that are exploited within the present social structure, and for whom existing services are either irrelevant or even harmful to their self-esteem.

Needs Assessment and Program Planning

The remaining three articles in this volume deal directly with needs assessment as a planning activity used to guide program development. The authors of these articles focus less on individual needs and more on the kinds of data most helpful to agencies planning prevention activities. As the reader will undoubtably discover, solutions depend greatly upon the nature of the problem being investigated. These articles discuss three problems: planning drug treatment services, developing primary prevention services for children, and coordinating resources among agencies to meet community needs.

Flaherty, Kotranski, and Fox faced the problem of how to best predict demand for drug treatment services. As experts in this field know, rates under treatment for drug use are highly volatile. In Philadelphia, between 1976 and 1977, there was a sharp and unexpected decline in the demand for services, underscoring the necessity of a more thorough understanding of the factors affecting community needs. The authors develop a measurement model with which to predict drug use rates and service demands within specific geographic areas. In doing so they explore with the reader the strengths and weaknesses of many different approaches including social area analysis, the use of archival data on criminal activity, and the identification of "copping" areas—street corners known for high rates of illicit drug traffic. Their integrative approach to the investigation of drug use and treatment needs is among the most comprehensive attempted.

Prevention activities for children are always at the cutting edge of the profession; no other target group has as much to gain or as much to lose. The identification of the needs for this group requires the utmost care; not only can children suffer from neglect of needed services, but ineffective services can also be harmful if, for example, a stigma is associated with them. Felner and Aber develop a strong case for the assessment of stressful circumstances to identify high risk children in place of parent-identified or school-identified problems. They argue that once a problem has been identified, it may already be too late for primary prevention activities. Their essay is sprinkled with real life examples of the practical and political problems as well as the conceptual issues involved in doing a truly prevention oriented need assessment. It is an excellent rhetorical companion for professionals concerned with meeting children's mental health needs preventatively.

The last paper in this group addresses the very sobering realities of diminishing agency resources. The authors, Meissen and Cipriani, present a method of systematically assessing the resources and needs of community agencies that can be used to identify gaps and redundancies in the existing service network. For them, needs assessment is a management tool that can be used to enhance resource exchanges among, within and between agencies. They propose collaborative strategies between agencies as a tonic for limited resources in place of the wasteful competition that has pervaded agency interrelations in recent years.

The articles in this volume demonstrate many innovative ways needs assessment can be used for prevention purposes. They emphasize that needs assessment can be applied to a variety of problems; that needs can be examined on an individual, organizational, and community level; and that theory, research, and action can walk hand-in-hand. Needs assessment plays an important role in the planning process and can be used to develop specific programs, aid in policy decisions, and provide valuable information for program evaluation efforts. While no panacea, it can make the winding and bumpy road to prevention much straighter and smoother.

Alex Zautra
Kenneth Bachrach

REFERENCES

Faris, R., & Dunham, H. *Mental disorders in urban areas.* Chicago: University of Chicago Press, 1939.

Leighton, D.C., Harding, J.S., Macklin, D.B., MacMillan, A.M., & Leighton, A.H. *The character of danger* (Vol. 3 of the Stirling County Study). New York: Basic Books, 1963.

Roueche, B. *Curiosities of medicine.* Boston: Little, Brown, 1958.

Shevky, E. & Bell, W. *Social area analysis.* Stanford: Stanford University Press, 1955.

Snow, J. *On the mode of communication of cholera.* London: Churchill, 1855. Reported in MacMahon, B., Puch, T.F., & Ipsen, J. *Epidemiologic Methods.* Boston: Little, Brown, 1960.

Strole, L., Langner, T.S., Michael, S.T., Opler, M.K., & Rennie, T.A.C. *Mental health in the metropolis: The Midtown Manhattan study* (Vol. I). New York: McGraw-Hill, 1962.

Warheit, G.J., Bell, R.A., & Schwab, J.J. *Planning for change: Needs assessment approaches.* Gainesville, FL: J. Hillis Miller Health Center, University of Florida, 1974.

Mental Health Needs Assessment Approaches: A Case for Applied Epidemiology

George J. Warheit
William A. Vega
Joanne Buhl-Auth

ABSTRACT. This paper briefly describes the political and social factors which have prompted the rapid development of needs assessment as a research activity. It also suggests reasons for the likelihood of continuing assessment mandates through the 1980s. The five most commonly employed needs assessment methodologies are outlined and a critique is offered for each. The major focus of the paper is on the development and uses of an applied epidemiologic survey assessment model which has been designed and tested extensively by the authors in a variety of geographic areas and agency settings. Illustrations of how field survey data can be presented for enumerating mental health needs are also presented.

The assessment of mental health needs as a scientific enterprise has emerged in relatively recent times. Its rapid development as a field of scientific inquiry can be attributed largely to federal statutes which have mandated that human service agencies receiving funds document the need for their services. In the mental health field, federal needs assessment mandates began with the 1963 legislation which established the comprehensive community mental health centers programs (PL 88-164); applicants were required to demonstrate a need for the services outlined in their construction and staffing grant requests. Inasmuch as the political climate was extremely favorable at the time and because funds for health and health related activities were being appropriated at record levels, the needs assessment sections of these applications were addressed most often in a

Reprints may be obtained from George J. Warheit, Department of Psychiatry, University of Florida, Gainesville, FL 32610.

9

perfunctory way. Within a relatively brief period of time, however, other legislation was enacted which specifically mandated more comprehensive needs documentation. For example, Public Law 89-749, passed in 1966, made explicit the expectation that human service agencies would identify and enumerate the need for their services and would organize their programs to meet those needs. The same intent is found in Public Law 93-64 which was enacted in 1975. Moreover, this law provided organizational structures, i.e., Health Systems Agencies, to facilitate and regulate the needs assessment process, particularly as it involved services and facilities. Public Law 94-63 (1975) also outlined a series of required planning and evaluation activities including needs assessment. Thus, between 1970 and 1980, the pressures exerted on publicly funded agencies to conduct needs assessments grew more intense and structured.

The social and political factors prompting these mandates are so complex that a detailed discussion of them is beyond the scope of this paper. A number of them are worth noting briefly, however. First, there was a dramatic alteration of the country's optimistic mood regarding the effectiveness of many of the social programs initiated during the 1960s. Changes in political ideologies, inflation, a general economic downturn, and the escalation of federally reimbursed health costs also contributed to the increased demands for accountability. Although the future of federal support for human services and regulations associated with that support is presently unclear, there is no reason to believe that the functions of needs assessment research will be diminished in the decade ahead. To the contrary, it is more logical to conclude that the importance of assessment research will increase as resources become more scarce. Greater accountability can be expected and, simultaneously, agencies will be compelled to maximize their efficiency and effectiveness as they endeavor to meet the service demands being imposed on them. This paper is written within the context of these perspectives and is offered as a tool for those who are seeking a scientifically rigorous and cost effective method of defining and enumerating the mental health needs of general populations. More specifically, this paper has three major purposes: (1) to describe and to critique briefly the most commonly used needs assessment techniques; (2) to outline in detail an extensively tested field survey assessment model; and (3) to present examples of how data from psychiatric epidemiologic field surveys can be used to assess the need for mental health services.

NEEDS ASSESSMENT TECHNIQUES

A number of needs assessment approaches have been used by mental health planners as they have attempted to meet the mandates prescribed by legislation. The senior author of this paper and his colleagues have described in detail five of the most frequently utilized ones (Warheit, Bell, & Schwab, 1977). These are: (1) the community forum; (2) the rates-under-treatment; (3) the key informant; (4) the social indicators; and (5) the field survey. Only a brief discussion and critique of the first four of these is presented; the major focus of this paper is on the field survey and its uses for assessment and planning.

Community Forums

One of the most commonly employed methods of assessing the need for mental health services has been the community forum. This approach typically consists of arranging public meetings during which community members are encouraged to express their beliefs regarding the need for differing types of programs. Occasionally, questionnaires are distributed and those present are requested to rank order the community's needs as they perceive them. More frequently, the data are gathered less formally through an open discussion of those present. After compiling the information generated by the forum, planners are presumably in a position to assess a community's needs and, ostensibly, to evaluate existing programs in the context of those needs. The findings are considered also to be of value in suggesting new areas for program development.

There are some benefits derived from conducting community forums. For example, the general public may develop a greater awareness of available services and the sponsoring agency is likely to become more visible in the community. The image of the agency may be improved as citizens sense its concern with their general well-being. Although community forums may produce some useful information and help create a positive image for the agency, there are a number of serious deficiencies which limit the validity of the needs assessment data obtained by them. One of these is related to the fact that forums can be dominated by organized lobbying-type groups which have the capacity to control meetings through sheer numbers, systematic organization, and/or through having a few prestigious and articulate persons represent their views. When this occurs, little useful needs data are likely to be secured by those conducting the forum. Another general criticism of the method is that it assumes those who are in the best position to express the varied needs within a community will attend and participate. This may not occur. The elderly, those with significant mental or physical health problems, and those with a wide range of other social and health needs often do not or cannot attend public meetings. Unless they are represented by others who serve as their proxies, their needs are not likely to be identified.

Community forums have additional limitations. One of the most potentially damaging of these is that they may increase the expectations on the part of an area's population regarding the development of programs which are not within an organization's domain or which cannot be addressed by the agency conducting the forum. When this occurs, latent frustrations within a community can emerge and be given a focus. As a consequence, officials may be compelled to defend aspects of their agency's mandates, priorities, and/or programs over which they have no choice or control. Thus, community forums may create and/or make manifest dissent and conflict, and those utilizing this method should consider this possible liability when weighing the relative merits of differing methodologies. In summary, forums are not usually representative of the general population within a community and the needs enumerated by them are often a reflection of the relative power of the persons and/or groups in attendance and their capacity to organize and direct the outcomes of the meeting. Moreover, forums can produce undesirable conflicts. Thus, while they may sometimes be useful, their overall value is open to serious questioning when they are evaluated as a needs assessment methodology.

Rates-Under-Treatment

A second widely used method of assessing mental health needs is the rates-under-treatment approach which relies on a descriptive enumeration of the clients utilizing the services of an agency. The basic premise of this method is that those who receive care represent the population in need. There are numerous limitations to this methodology. Most notably, there is an overwhelming body of data which has shown that many persons in serious need of mental health services do not receive them. For example, the "Task Panel Report on the Nature and Scope of Mental Health Problems in the United

States,'' a subsection of the President's Commission Report (1978), indicated that:

> Only about one-fourth of those suffering from a clinically sig-
> nificant disorder have been in treatment. The median propor-
> tion of true cases ever in treatment among those suffering from
> all psychotic disorders is 59.7% based on evidence from seven
> studies, and the corresponding rate for schizophrenia alone is
> 81.1% based on six studies. . . . These figures . . . mean that
> two out of every five persons with psychosis and one out of
> every five with schizophrenia have never received treat-
> ment. . . . Only 35% of those currently suffering from a ma-
> jor depression were receiving any general medical treatment
> and only 30% received psychiatric or mental health treatment
> in the year before the disabling episode. (p. 22)

This strong evidence of underutilization of services reflects the most significant weakness of the rates-under-treatment method. A more appropriate function of treatment data is in the evaluation phase of the planning process where they can be employed to make judgments about the outreach of an agency within the context of previously established needs data. However, to reiterate, as a method it does not provide a sound basis for assessing mental health needs.

Key Informants

A third methodology used extensively in conducting needs assess-
ment research is the key informant one (cf. Buhl-Auth, Note 1). This method relies on responses from individuals who are assumed, on the basis of their personal or professional characteristics, to have knowledge of a community's mental health needs. Two of the prag-
matic values of this method are the conceptual simplicity of its design and its relative inexpensiveness. Its value is expanded when the key informants are brought together to discuss their individual and collective assessments. This is especially true when the respondents are selected so as to represent both the public and private sectors. These discussions can increase an individual agency's awareness of its role as perceived by significant others and, in addition, how its programs are interrelated within the broader ser-
vice context. These outcomes may be of sufficient interest to justify

conducting a key informant study. At the same time, those considering its use should be aware of its limitations. These have been detailed by this author and his colleagues (Warheit, Buhl, & Bell,
1978), who conducted a multimethod needs assessment project in a
midwestern city. They found that at a global level informants could
correctly distinguish between the geographic areas of greatest and
least need. At the same time, the informants were markedly divided
in their assessments of need in three other subareas within the community. More importantly, they were not successful in their efforts
to estimate the prevalence or magnitude of specific problems within
or between any of the five geographic subdivisions of the county.
Other researchers have encountered methodological difficulties.
The staff of an agency working in a southeastern planning area
found that establishing a scientifically defensible sampling frame,
identifying informants, and getting adequate response rates posed
major difficulties in interpreting the findings (North Central
Georgia Health Systems Agency Report on Key Informants, 1979).
On the basis of these and other research efforts, our conclusion is
that the key informant method does not offer much promise as a
scientifically rigorous approach to the identifying of specific needs
among differing subpopulations within communities.

Social Indicators Method

Social indicators analysis has been used extensively as an assessment strategy by mental health planners. This method relies on secondary data sources containing items which have a presumed or
demonstrated association with mental health problems and/or treatment (Warheit, Holzer, & Robbins, 1979). The most widely known
social indicators model in the mental health field is the Mental
Health Demographic Profile System (MHDPS). This methodology
was developed by researchers at the National Institute of Mental
Health and is based on a large number of items drawn from the U.S.
Census (Rosen, Goldsmith, & Redick, 1979). The system arranges
its indicators within several broad content areas such as general
population data, social and economic status, race-ethnicity, famil-
ism, life cycle stages, and populations at high risk. Norms which
permit one to compare local community mental health center catchment areas with all other tracted catchment areas in the United
States are also provided by the system. The MHDPS is extremely
useful in generating a broad social and demographic overview of a

community and it has great utility for all mental health planners when used for this purpose. In addition, the data produced by it can be used effectively to identify subpopulations whose characteristics are commonly associated with known levels of need for mental health care.

As an assessment strategy, the system does have a number of limitations inherent in it. One of these is that the indicators are, at best, proxies for mental health problems and as a consequence they do not provide specific information on the levels or kinds of needs in a community. In addition, the data are presented as demographic and ecological aggregates. This fact dictates caution in their use so as to avoid ecological fallacies. The lack of specificity and the aggregated character of the data confounds the interpretation of social indicators findings. These difficulties are exacerbated further when the census data are old or when they are not available for a given planning area.

These four methods of assessing mental health needs have been widely used and each has value when the objectives of the research do not require a precise enumeration of mental health problems. At the same time, all of these approaches have theoretical and methodological inadequacies which limit the use of the findings derived from them. For this reason, those wishing scientifically rigorous information regarding the prevalence of mental health problems in an area must depend on data obtained by means of field surveys conducted with carefully drawn statistical probability samples of the general population.

ASSESSING MENTAL HEALTH NEEDS:
AN EXAMPLE OF APPLIED EPIDEMIOLOGY

The authors of this paper, along with a large number of colleagues, have been involved in testing each of the five methodologies outlined by Warheit, Bell, & Schwab (1977). This testing has occurred in a variety of agencies and in different regions of the United States. A comprehensive monograph summarizing these efforts is forthcoming (Warheit & Buhl-Auth, Note 2). On the basis of this extensive work, we have concluded that the needs assessment data produced by scientifically designed and implemented field surveys have the greatest overall value for mental health planning. The reasons for this conclusion involve these considerations.

The most important advantage of a field survey is that it is the only method which can access directly a representative sample of the population whose needs are being assessed. All of the other methods have inherent weaknesses as far as the representativeness of their findings is concerned. By focusing on the general population and relying on statistical probability sampling procedures, investigators are able to determine the randomness of their sample and, in turn, to defend the generalizability of their findings. No other assessment methodology permits researchers to address these important scientific issues.

Field surveys have additional scientific advantages. One of these is that the findings derived from probability samples are more amenable to tests for validity and reliability and can be tested more appropriately for statistical significance. Another advantage is that they can be designed to identify the specific needs and service patterns of the general populations and of most subpopulations living in a planning area. All of the other approaches rely on unobtrusive indicators and/or proxy measures of a population's mental health needs. As a consequence, non-survey methods cannot provide scientific data on the specific kinds of needs prevalent in a population and neither can they produce precise information on the varying magnitude of needs except in general, categorical ways. For these reasons surveys provide data of greater value for planning purposes than the alternative approaches.

This value is especially evident when the findings are being considered as a basis for making program and/or policy changes in an organization. The authors, in numerous agency settings, have been compelled to defend the data generated by differing types of assessment research. These demands are most rigorously expressed when the results call for program re-evaluation and/or changes. In these instances, without exception, the representativeness of the sample and the validity and reliability of the findings are challenged. When the results, conclusions, and implications of a needs assessment project can be defended on the basis of their scientific merit, the possibility of program change is enhanced greatly. Thus, the basic objective of assessment research, that is, the identification and enumeration of needs and the translation of this needs information into program modifications, is best accomplished by carefully conceived and conducted field surveys. This conclusion is not intended to discredit the other methods; it is offered to put them within a general comparative context. As detailed in a forthcoming monograph (Warheit & Buhl-Auth, Note 2), all of the approaches have their individual advantages; and they have been found to be of greatest utility when aspects of all of them are employed in a sequential, integrated, systemic fashion.

The Background of Field Surveys
as an Assessment Methodology

Interest in psychiatric epidemiology was intensified following World War II as data from the national selective service indicated that mental health problems accounted for a large percentage of those rejected for military duty. These selective service data, reinforced by other factors, most notably the development of psychotropic medications, were highly instrumental in the enactment of the 1963 legislation which established the community mental health centers program (PL 88-164). In turn, these two factors, i.e., the selective service data and the community mental health centers program, were the historical antecedents of the public laws mandating needs assessment as a condition for federal funding. As planners and administrators reviewed the available assessment methodologies, they tended to discount field surveys on the grounds that they were too complex and costly. Moreover, psychiatric epidemiology as a field of scientific inquiry was changing rapidly as investigators altered their data sources from treatment records to information secured from probability samples of the general population. And, overall, the state of the art of psychiatric epidemiology had not yet reached the level of sophistication whereby its methods could be employed by nonprofessional researchers for needs assessment purposes.

The early post World War II epidemiological studies typically determined global mental disorders by means of brief screening instruments, including scales and indexes. These measures were characteristically tested for content reliability by standard statistical procedures while their validity was established by psychiatric judges and/or comparative analyses with patient subsamples. The design, methods, theoretical assumptions, and findings from these surveys have been reported extensively in the literature (cf. Dohrenwend & Dohrenwend, 1969; Dohrenwend, Gould, Link, Neugebauer, & Wunsch-Hitzig, 1981; Langner & Michael, 1963; Leighton, Harding, & Macklin, 1963; Srole, Langner, & Michael, 1962). While most of the studies conducted in the 1950s and 1960s sought to establish global rates of psychiatric impairment (Leighton et al., 1963; Srole et al., 1962) using brief screening instruments, the research of Warheit, Schwab, and others centered more on determining the rates of specific symptoms, syndromes, and related dysfunctions, e.g., depression, anxiety, cognitive impairment, and general psychopathology (Schwab, Bell, Warheit, & Schwab, 1979; Schwab, McGinnis, & Warheit, 1970; Vega, 1981; Warheit, Holzer, Bell, & Arey, 1976; Warheit, Holzer, & Schwab, 1973).

At present, the Division of Biometry and Epidemiology of the National Institute of Mental Health is funding five large scale, long term Epidemiologic Catchment Area projects (ECAs) in different regions of the United States. These have been designed to enumerate the prevalence of many of the types of psychiatric disorders outlined in the Diagnostic and Statistical Manual of the American Psychiatric Association (1980). The purposes and scope of these projects cannot be discussed fully within the limitations of this paper. They are mentioned because they are the most sophisticated epidemiologic studies ever conducted and, further, they represent an extension of the interests which prompted the post World War II efforts. Those interested will find a useful description of the ECA program in a publication of Eaton, Regier, Locke, and Taube (1981). The core instrument being used to gather the psychiatric prevalence data in the ECA projects is the Diagnostic Interview Schedule (DIS). Developed under the auspices of the Division of Biometry and Epidemiology of the National Institute of Mental Health, the instrument is being widely tested by several different research groups. The results of these tests are now beginning to be published and it appears that the instrument will be valuable for researchers enumerating the prevalence and distribution of specific psychiatric disorders in the general population (Robins, Helzer, Croughan, & Ratcliff, 1981). The potential planning value of the findings produced by these projects is tremendous. Regrettably, these data will not be available for mental health planning uses in the near future. For this reason, we have continued to test and refine a field survey model for needs assessment purposes. We consider this model to be an applied epidemiologic one since it emerged from our earlier basic research.

Background of an Applied Epidemiologic Assessment Model

The survey model we are going to describe has been employed to secure needs data on 12,001 persons living in different regions of the United States. These needs assessment surveys have been completed by researchers representing a variety of organizations including universities, state and county departments of mental health, and local community mental health centers. A listing of the research sites, year conducted, sample sizes, and principal investigators is found in Table 1. All projects employed a common core of assessment and services utilization items as well as others designed to answer questions of interest to the individual investigators. The development and testing of all aspects of the survey model and many

Table 1

Research Sites, Sample Sizes and Principal Investigators of Projects

Using Field Survey Assessment Model* Total $\underline{N}$ = 12,001

Location	Year Conducted	Sample Size	Principal Invest.
Florida	1969-73	4,506	John Schwab George Warheit Roger Bell
Kentucky	1974-75	1,078	Roger Bell Martin Sundell John Schwab
California Mexican-American/Anglo	1980	1,345	William Vega Kenneth Meinhardt
Guamanian	1980	312	David Shimizu
Mexican Immigrants	1981	150	Luz Fernandez Pieda Garcia Sylvia Tello
Nebraska	1981	1,810	Peter Beeson
Ohio Northwest Study	1980	1,728	Richard Hunter Rick Naida
South Central	1980	1,072	Mary Stefl

*The senior author of this paper was either a co-principal

investigator or active consultant on all of the projects.

of the findings accruing from its use have been reported in the literature and, therefore, will not be detailed here (Schwab, Bell, Warheit, & Schwab, 1979; Schwab, McGinnis, & Warheit, 1970; Vega, 1981; Warheit, 1979; Warheit, Holzer, Bell, & Arey, 1976; Warheit, Holzer, & Schwab, 1973; Warheit, Vega, Meinhardt, & Shimizu, 1982; Warheit & Buhl-Auth, Note 2; Kuldau, Warheit, & Holzer, Note 3; Warheit, Note 4; Warheit & Buhl-Auth, Note 5). The purposes of this paper do require a brief synopsis of the development and testing of the psychiatric scales included in all of the surveys inasmuch as they generate the data by which mental health needs are identified. As such, these measures constitute the central component of our applied epidemiologic method.

The survey assessment approach we have developed calls for the securing of information by means of a structured interview schedule. The various schedules have been found to take approximately 20-30 minutes to complete. They have been administered in person and over the telephone with equal success. The core of all the schedules has consisted of five psychiatric symptom and dysfunction scales which were developed by factor and principal components analysis. The scales tap these symptom and dysfunctions: depression, anxiety, psychosocial dysfunction, cognitive impairment, and general psychopathology. The reliability of these measures was tested using a method developed by Cronbach (1951) and modified by Bornstedt (1969). These tests showed that all scales had coefficients of reliability above .70 in all survey settings. The scales were tested for content and construct validity in several ways, the details of which can be only briefly sketched here. These were as follows.

Clinical judgments were made whereby three psychiatrists, independently and blinded, assessed the mental health status of 362 psychiatric patients and 432 respondents from community samples. The results showed that the patients had significantly higher scores on all scales than did the community respondents. In addition, the level of need for services, as assessed by the psychiatrists, was significantly associated with the scale scores of both the patient and non-patient samples. It is important to mention that the psychiatrist judges did not have access to any of the scores for either group (Schwab et al., 1979; Warheit & Buhl-Auth, Note 5).

A second test for validity included a follow-up study of 567 persons who had been interviewed three years earlier. The findings on validity showed that the majority of those with scale scores one or more standard deviations above the mean for the entire sample at the time of their initial interview had disproportionately high scores at the follow-up. Among other things, this finding validated the stability of the symptom/dysfunction patterns over time (Schwab et al., 1979; Warheit, 1979).

A third validity study consisted of scale score comparisons between a psychiatric inpatient sample, $N = 256$, and respondents from a field survey sample, $N = 1645$ (Kuldau, Warheit, & Holzer, Note 3). The psychiatric inpatient sample was selected from cases being treated by two community mental health centers located in the same area as the respondents chosen for the field survey. Patients diagnosed as being mentally retarded, suffering from organic brain syndromes, and/or having alcohol or drug disorders were excluded from the sample. The patients included in the study were administered the same symptom and dysfunction scales which had been given to the community sample. In addition to the psychiatric scales, respondents in the community sample were asked a series of questions related to their personal life experiences in the preceding year, and in the previous three years. Using the life experience data, a panel of experts identified ten factors which they judged to be related to the need for mental health services. These factors included life crisis events, e.g., the death of a child, spouse, or other family member, marital separation or divorce, serious health problems or disabilities, and the utilization of health services. The number of events for each of the respondents in the community sample was enumerated. Then, this sample was divided into four groups on the basis of the number of risk factors reported by them. These groups were: (1) no risk factors; (2) 1-2 risk factors; (3) 3-5 risk factors; and (4) 5 or more risk factors. The mean psychiatric scale scores for the various risk groups from the community sample were then compared with the mean scores of the patient sample. The analysis indicated that the scores of the patient group were significantly higher, $p < .05$, than those of the no risk and 1-2 risk factor groups on all scales. By contrast, the mean scores of the 5 or more risk factor group and the patient groups were not significantly different from one another on any of the scales. The analysis also indicated that the mean psychiatric scale scores of the lower two and higher two risk groups were significantly different from one another at the $p < .05$ level or greater. This study further validated the symptom and dysfunction scales as criteria for distinguishing between the mental health needs of general populations.

The final test of validity for the psychiatric scales consisted of an analytic procedure which compared the scale scores of respondents with a total of 59 other variables included in the survey. The 59 factors chosen for this analysis represented conditions or behaviors which have known associations with mental health problems, e.g., inability to get or keep a job; a history of interpersonal conflicts with disruptive consequences; frequent changes of residence; social isolation; excessive alcohol or drug use; suicidal ideation; and negative self-perceptions of physical health, mental health, and personal well-being. The associations between high scale scores and all 59 of these factors were statistically significant at the .05 level or greater (Warheit, Note 4).

The findings from these extensive tests have indicated that the symptom and dysfunction scales developed to assess mental health needs are reliable and valid measures.

The Uses of Field Survey Data
for Assessing Mental Health Needs

One of the characteristics that surveys have is that the data from them are amenable to a great many modes of presentation. The authors have used a variety of standard techniques for describing field survey findings, e.g., bar and line graphs, percentage distributions, and transparent overlays which show the patterns of differing levels and kinds of needs among a population. They have also used a variety of complex statistical approaches such as factor analysis, cluster analysis, and confirmatory factor procedures. Each of these has some intrinsic value for presenting assessment data but the use of multiple methods for detailing the findings is preferred in most cases. Of course, the method or combination of methods selected to present research results depends on the objectives of the research, the nature of the data, and the audience being addressed. Even a brief description of the numerous techniques which can be employed for analyzing, displaying, and communicating survey derived assessment data is beyond the scope and intent of this paper. Rather than attempting an exhaustive description of this very important set of activities, the focus is on procedures we have developed and found to be most useful when presenting quantitative assessment information. Once again, the survey model detailed above serves as a guide for the discussion.

Before proceeding, it is crucial to make explicit one of the most basic assumptions underlying our research, since it has a powerful influence on the ways the data are presented. The assumption is this: there is a relationship between the level of psychiatric symptomatology and associated dysfunctions and the magnitude of need for mental health services. This position was supported by the extensive validity studies outlined above. The analyses which tested the relationships between the symptom and dysfunction scale scores and 59 separate variables known from the clinical and epidemiological literature to be highly associated with mental health problems were of particular value in developing many of our data presentation methods. In addition to the formal tests for validity, it is logical to conclude on the basis of face validity alone that those with the most intense symptom and related patterns of dysfunction are in the greatest need for services.

One of the techniques developed for analyzing and presenting survey data for assessment purposes was constructed as follows. The mean scores for the entire sample were calculated for each of the symptom/dysfunction scales. They were also computed for the major social and demographic subgroups in the community. The results of these analyses are reported in Table 2 under the heading labelled *mean.*

A review of Table 2 shows that the mean score on the scale designed to measure depressive symptomatology was 14.28 for the sample as a whole. The possible range of scores on this scale is 0-72. A further examination of the data reveals that some subgroups had higher mean depression scale scores than others. Those separated and those in the lowest socioeconomic status group, as determined by an index combining education, occupation, and income, had the highest scores in the sample. It can also be seen that blacks had higher mean scores than whites and that females had higher scores than males. This tabulation requires very little mathematical expertise to construct. If nothing more than this calculation of the mean scale scores were done, planners/administrators would still be able to identify from this table the differential levels of depressive symptomatology among subgroups in their communities.

By itself, the presentation of mean scale scores for differing groups has important implications for planning and evaluation. This value is increased by determining the statistical significance of the mean score differences between groups. The most frequently utilized methods for doing this are *t*-tests and analyses of variance (ANOVA). These procedures are outlined in most elementary

TABLE 2

THE DISTRUBUTION OF DEPRESSION SCORES AND PERCENT
SCORING ONE OR MORE STANDARD DEVIATIONS ABOVE THE MEAN
BY RACE, SEX, AGE, MARITAL STATUS, SES GROUPS

	N	Mean	SD	Sig.	% High
TOTAL	4202	14.28	9.60	---	15.9
RACE					
White	3469	13.61	9.23	t=10.17	13.9
Black	707	17.59	10.71	***	26.0
SEX					
Male	1807	12.51	8.88	t=10.58	10.9
Female	2395	15.63	9.90	***	19.6
AGE					
<20	197	15.78	8.98		15.2
20-29	907	14.24	8.39	ANOVA	12.2
30-39	631	13.99	9.28	F=2.53*	15.2
40-49	639	14.58	10.06	df=6,4187	18.5
50-59	621	15.02	10.61	R=-0.0281	19.5
60-69	624	13.92	9.98		16.3
70+	575	13.43	9.78		15.4
MARITAL STATUS					
Single	527	15.54	8.98		15.0
Married	2765	13.07	8.98	ANOVA	12.5
Widowed	535	16.25	10.51	F=45.81***	24.1
Separated	130	22.15	11.60	df=4,4178	43.1
Divorced	226	16.41	10.46	R=0.1085	22.1
SES					
1. 0-19 (low)	432	19.47	11.92		35.2
2. 20-39	798	16.59	10.76	ANOVA	23.9
3. 40-59	933	14.54	9.55	F=73.02***	15.9
4. 60-79	1246	12.29	7.99	df=4,4194	9.6
5. 80-99 (high)	790	11.96	7.41	R=-0.2469	7.2

  * p<.05
 ** p<.01
*** p<.005

statistics books and they can be calculated by hand although the process would be tedious and take a long period of time when used with large data sets. When the sample sizes and the number of variables are not too large, minicomputers along with the appropriate software can be utilized to accomplish these procedures. The results produced show the statistical magnitude of scale score differences which at face value may not appear to be very great. The statistical significances of the mean score differences for the groups described in Table 2 are found under the heading labelled *sig.* (significance).

Two additional categories of information are shown in Table 2 under the headings *SD,* which represents standard deviation, and *percent high.* The data presented in these columns were established as follows. First, as noted, the mean scores were calculated. The next step consisted of determining the standard deviations for each group. This procedure, which is also outlined in most introductory statistics books, describes the fluctuation of individual scale scores as they occur above and below the mean score for the entire group. When a population is "normally" distributed in a statistical sense, approximately two-thirds of all individuals will have scores which fall between one standard deviation below and one standard deviation above the mean for the total group. The mean depression score for the sample described in Table 2 is 14.28 and the standard deviation is 9.60. This suggests, assuming the sample was "normally" distributed, that two-thirds of those surveyed will have scores which range from 4.68 to 23.88. Since one of our fundamental assumptions was that those with the highest scores would be those in greatest need, attention was given to those with scores above the mean for the sample. More specifically, we isolated those subgroups whose scores were one or more standard deviations above the sample mean and present this information under the heading, *percent high.*

The application of statistical normative methods as described enables one to display in a dramatic way the differential depression scores for the sample's social and demographic subgroups. For example, 43.1% of those maritally separated had scores one or more standard deviations above the sample mean. Other subgroups with high percentages of their members one or more standard deviations above the sample mean were blacks (26.0%), the widowed (24.1%), and those in the lowest socioeconomic group (35.2%). To reiterate, this method of analyzing and presenting data enables one to identify the subpopulations in a community with the greatest levels of specific symptomatology/dysfunctions.

The techniques just described were followed for the other scales included in the interview schedule. After the means, standard deviations, and percent high were derived for all of the scales, an additional step was completed. The social and demographic subgroups in the sample were placed into one of four categories as dictated by their scale scores. These were: no scales high; one to two scales high; three to four scales high; and five scales high. The data generated by these procedures are reported in Table 3. The rationale for arranging the sample into these four categories is twofold. First,

TABLE 3

PERCENT SCORING 1 OR MORE STANDARD DEVIATIONS ABOVE THE MEAN
ON FIVE SYMPTOM/DYSFUNCTION SCALES BY SOCIODEMOGRAPHIC GROUPS

		Scales High			
	N	None %	1-2 %	3-4 %	5 %
TOTAL	3540	60.3	27.5	9.9	2.4
RACE					
White	2909	61.5	27.6	8.9	1.9
Black	609	53.7	27.1	14.6	4.6
SEX					
Male	1538	65.0	26.7	6.2	2.1
Female	2002	56.7	28.0	12.6	2.6
RACE/SEX					
White Male	1277	65.6	27.3	5.6	1.5
White Female	1632	58.3	27.8	11.6	2.3
Black Male	247	60.7	23.9	10.1	5.3
Black Female	362	48.9	29.3	17.7	4.1
AGE					
18-19	186	51.1	36.0	11.8	1.1
20-29	810	59.6	29.4	9.0	2.0
30-39	557	63.0	24.6	9.3	3.1
40-49	533	62.9	25.0	9.2	3.0
50-59	504	57.9	28.2	11.3	2.6
60-69	502	62.0	25.9	10.0	2.2
70+	442	59.7	28.1	10.2	2.0
MARITAL STATUS					
Single	470	55.3	31.9	11.3	1.5
Married	2304	64.4	26.0	7.6	2.0
Widowed	430	52.8	30.2	14.9	2.1
Separated	116	37.9	26.7	25.9	9.5
Divorced	205	56.6	27.8	11.2	4.4
SOCIOECONOMIC STATUS					
Lowest 1	318	39.0	31.4	23.9	5.7
2	660	54.7	27.6	12.9	4.8
3	836	58.5	28.8	11.1	1.6
4	1052	67.7	25.0	5.8	1.5
Highest 5	673	66.7	27.6	4.9	0.7

the comprehensive studies completed to evaluate the content and construct validity of the psychiatric scales revealed distinct relationships between the composite scale scores of respondents and their levels of psychopathology. It was found, for example, that there were statistically significant relationships between the scales high categories and all 59 factors associated with the need for mental health services. These analyses, along with the other validity studies, justify the four group categorization.

A second reason for developing the four scales high categories is a practical one. Mental health needs are complex, multidimensional constructs and, as a consequence, the information required to identify the various elements within them is very extensive. For the presentation of assessment findings, this information must be condensed before it can be effectively communicated. We believe the development of the scales high categories is an efficient as well as a valid method for reducing large quantities of data into manageable proportions for presentation and planning functions.

A review of the information found in Table 3 reveals that about two-thirds of the sample (60.3%) scored in the normal ranges on all five scales. As one reads down the column labelled *none,* wide disparaties are seen. White males had the largest percentage of respondents in the no scales high group (65.6%); the separated had the lowest percentage (37.9%). Other groups with small percentages of their members in the no scales high category were black females (48.9%) and those in the lowest socioeconomic status groups (39.0%). This information illustrates clearly the differential distribution of psychiatric symptoms/dysfunctions, i.e., mental health needs, among and between the various social and demographic groups in this sample. An analysis of the three to four scales high and the five scales high categories shows similar, but not always identical, patterns. The separated, blacks, those in the lowest socioeconomic status groups, the widowed, and the divorced had the highest percentages of their cohorts in these scales high categories. Once again, these data identify the varying need levels of those in the community from which the sample was drawn, and they do so in a succinct and easily understandable manner.

A final way we have employed psychiatric epidemiologic survey data for assessment purposes has consisted of establishing rates estimates for differing levels of need and for varying social and demographic subgroups (Warheit & Buhl-Auth, Note 2). This method involved the following steps.

1. The scales high categories from Table 3 were re-defined as no scales high—no need; one to two scales high—low need; three to four scales high—moderate need; and five scales high—high need. These new categories were developed following an analysis of the reliability and validity studies and from a concurrent review of the findings produced by several of the field surveys (Warheit & Buhl-Auth, Note 2). The no need group, i.e., those scoring in the normal ranges on all scales, were not considered further in this particular analytic procedure.

2. The percentages of respondents in each of the newly defined needs groups were converted into rates per hundred by moving the decimal point two places to the left. Then a mental health need rates table was prepared. These rates are presented in Table 4.

3. An enumeration of the total number of persons in each of the differing social and demographic groups in the planning area was obtained from reports of the U.S. Bureau of the Census.

4. The number of persons in the subgroups was then multiplied by the need rates for that subgroup. These data were used to prepare a matrix which displayed the number of persons with low, moderate and high needs in each social and demographic subpopulation. They were also employed to calculate and present the total number in all need groups.

The method described in these four steps identifies the number of persons in an area in terms of their relative need for mental services and it does so within the context of their social and demographic characteristics. By providing the number of people in need and the level of their need, these data are of great value for meeting assessment objectives.

It is recognized that the process of applying rates tables in the field of psychiatric epidemiology has limitations inherent in it. The need rates we have developed and employed in constructing Table 4 closely parallel the morbidity tables developed by epidemiologists working in other fields. The central problems associated with the development and application of morbidity rates, i.e., needs rates, in the mental health area have their origins in the issues of definition, that is, what constitutes a need, and in measurement, that is, how can those needs be measured reliably and validly. We do not presume to have definitively addressed the theoretical and methodological issues underlying these central problems. At the same time, all aspects of the applied epidemiologic assessment model described in this paper have been tested repeatedly and the model has been

Table 4

Estimated Rates of Need for Mental Health Services Based on

Psychiatric Symptom Score Distributions

	Low	Moderate	High
Total Population	.275	.098	.024
Race:			
White	.276	.089	.019
Nonwhite	.271	.146	.046
Sex:			
Male	.268	.062	.021
Female	.280	.126	.026
Race/Sex:			
White Male	.273	.056	.015
White Female	.278	.116	.023
Nonwhite Male	.239	.102	.053
Nonwhite Female	.293	.176	.041
Age:			
18-19	.360	.118	.011
20-29	.294	.090	.020
30-39	.246	.094	.031
40-49	.249	.092	.032
50-59	.281	.113	.026
60-69	.259	.100	.022
70+	.281	.101	.020
Education (yrs. completed):			
Elementary 0-4	.284	.214	.065
5-8	.285	.128	.029
High School 1-3	.280	.127	.042
4	.253	.077	.016
College 1-3	.307	.074	.012
4+	.259	.035	.008
Marital Status:			
Single	.319	.112	.015
Married	.260	.076	.020
Widowed	.302	.149	.021
Separated	.267	.259	.095
Divorced	.278	.112	.044

used successfully by planners in a variety of agency and geographic settings. Nonetheless, we would caution against the indiscriminant application of the needs rates we have developed. When considering their use, one must keep in mind that the scales on which these rates are based must be tested for reliability and validity in the areas where they are going to be applied. The failure to do this greatly diminishes the scientific defensibility of the results and in the process seriously limits their utility. The work we and our colleagues around the country have already completed greatly reduces the tasks associated with the development, testing, and application of these rates. But, to reiterate, before using them for making needs projections they should be tested with subsamples of the population in the planning area where the assessment is being conducted.

The tasks related to completing validity and reliability studies require methodological and statistical expertise. Statistical probability samples of the general population or of previously identified subsamples must be drawn and those selected must be interviewed in person or by phone. In addition, patient samples need to be interviewed for the purpose of establishing validity; such samples are often available from local mental health agencies. The size of the samples required to complete the reliability and validity studies need not be nearly as large as those described in this paper and most of the other instrumentation is already in place. Our belief is that the research required to test the scales which serve as the basis of our needs rates can be economically and successfully completed by most human service agencies in this country. When the skills required to complete the necessary tasks are not available among the personnel of an agency, they can be secured from other public and private organizations such as planning councils, state or county health agencies, and academic institutions.

It is reasonable to conclude that the ECA projects and other research using the DIS will in the future produce valid and reliable data on the prevalence of specific disorders for subpopulations residing in different areas of the United States. When this occurs, it will be possible to determine the rates for these disorders. And, hopefully, the DIS will be used frequently enough in the years ahead to justify the application of these rates to determine the needs for specific treatment programs. This does not mean to imply, of course, that the DIS resolves the issues of etiology. It is primarily a system of classification and as such does not directly address the fundamental questions regarding cause. Nonetheless, it represents a significant step forward in the field of epidemiology and its use holds much promise for the development of applied epidemiology as an assessment modality.

SUMMARY

Legislative requirements to document the need for mental health services will probably continue in some form in the decade ahead. This paper was written within the context of this belief and is offered to assist those engaged in planning and evaluating mental health programs. The methodologies described have been tested extensively by the authors in a variety of agencies and in differing regions of the United States. Their experience has shown them that the field survey is the most scientifically defensible assessment methodology available, and for this reason they have developed and tested a survey model for use by agencies with limited resources. The parameters of this model and data from a project based on it were presented to illustrate some of the ways survey data can be obtained and used for assessment purposes. And, the potential value of current developments in psychiatric research as represented by the ECA projects was discussed in the context of the future uses of applied epidemiology.

In summary, the authors believe that needs assessment research, especially when conducted with rigorously developed and tested models, regardless of their type, affords agencies with an extremely valuable mechanism for identifying the mental health problems of persons in their service areas. Without such assessments, services cannot be rationally planned. And, in the absence of careful planning, limited resources may be inefficiently expended and, most importantly, the needs of those experiencing mental health problems may not be addressed.

REFERENCE NOTES

1. Buhl-Auth, J. *The use of key informants to assess mental health needs* (Technical report). Gainesville, FL: University of Florida, Department of Psychiatry Research Unit, 1982.

2. Warheit, G., & Buhl-Auth, J. *An integrated approach to needs assessment research* (Technical report). Gainesville, FL: University of Florida, Department of Psychiatry Research Unit, forthcoming, 1983.

3. Kuldau, J., Warheit, G., & Holzer, C. *Developing risk analysis with community and patient populations* (Technical report). Gainesville, FL: University of Florida, Department of Psychiatry Research Unit, 1976.
4. Warheit, G. *An assessment of the need for mental health services in the state of California* (Technical report). Sacramento, CA: California Department of Mental Health, 1981.
5. Warheit, G., & Buhl-Auth, J. *The Florida health study scales: Their development and testing* (Technical report). Gainesville, FL: University of Florida, Department of Psychiatry Research Unit, 1982.

REFERENCES

Bohrnstedt, G. A quick method for determining the reliability and validity of multiple item scales. *American Sociological Review,* 1969, *34,* 542-548.
Cronbach, D. *Essentials of psychological testing.* New York: Harper, 1951.
Diagnostic and statistical manual III of the American Psychiatric Association. Washington, D.C.: American Psychiatric Association, 1980.
Dohrenwend, B. P., & Dohrenwend, B. S. *Social status and psychological disorder: A causal inquiry.* New York: Wiley Interscience, 1969.
Dohrenwend, B. P., Dohrenwend, B. S., Gould, M., Link, B., Neugebauer, R., & Wunsch-Hitzig, R. *Mental illness in the United States.* New York: Praeger Scientific, 1981.
Eaton, W., Regier, D., Locke, B., & Taube, C. The epidemiologic catchment area program of the National Institute of Mental Health. *Public Health Reports,* 1981, *96,* 319-325.
Langner, T., & Michael S. *Life stress and mental illness.* New York: Free Press of Glencoe, 1963.
Leighton, D., Harding, J., & Macklin, D. *The character of danger.* New York: Free Press of Glencoe, 1963.
MacMillan, A. The health opinion survey: Technique for estimating prevalence of psychoneurotic and related types of disorders in communities. *Psychological Reports,* 1957, *3,* 325-329.
Mental health status indicators. Atlanta, GA: North Central Georgia Health Systems Agency, October, 1979.
Report of the president's commission on mental health: Scope of the problem. Washington, D.C.: U.S. Government Printing Office, 1978.
Robins, L., Helzer, J., Croughan, J., & Ratcliff, K. National institute of mental health diagnostic interview schedule. *Archives of General Psychiatry,* 1981, *38,* 381-389.
Rosen, B., Goldsmith, H., & Redlick, R. Demographic and social indicators from the U.S. census of population and housing: Uses for mental health planning in small areas. *World Health Organization Quarterly,* 1979, *32*(1), 11-101.
Schwab, J., Bell, R., Warheit, G., & Schwab, R. *Social order and mental health.* New York: Bruner-Mazel, 1979.
Schwab, J., McGinnis, N., & Warheit, G. Toward a social psychiatric definition of impairment. *British Journal of Psychiatry,* 1970, *1,* 41-47.
Srole, L., Langner, T., & Michael, S. *Mental health in the metropolis: The midtown Manhattan study.* New York: McGraw-Hill, 1962.
Vega, W. Defining Hispanic high risk groups: Targeting populations for health promotion. *Hispanic natural support systems.* Sacramento, CA: California Department of Mental Health, 1981.
Warheit, G. Life events, coping, stress and depressive symptomatology. *American Journal of Psychiatry,* 1979, *136,* 502-507.
Warheit, G., Bell, R., & Schwab, J. *Needs assessment approaches: Concepts and methods* (DHEW Publication No. ADM 77-472). Washington, D.C.: U.S. Government Printing Office, 1977.

Warheit, G., Buhl-Auth, J., & Bell, R. A critique of social indicators analysis and key informants surveys as needs assessment methods. *Evaluation and Program Planning*, 1978, *1*, 239-247.
Warheit, G., Holzer, C., Bell, R., & Arey, S. Sex, marital status and mental health: A reappraisal. *Social Forces*, 1976, *3*, 223-237.
Warheit, G., Holzer, C., & Robbins, L. Social indicators and mental health planning: An empirical case study. *Community Mental Health Journal*, 1979, *15*, 94-103.
Warheit, G., Holzer, C., & Schwab, J. An analysis of social class and racial differences in depressive symptomatology: A community study. *Journal of Health and Social Behavior*, 1973, *4*, 291-299.
Warheit, G., Vega, W., Meinhardt, K., & Shimizu, D. Interpersonal coping networks and mental health problems among four race-ethnic groups. *Journal of Community Psychology*, 1982, *10*, 312-324.

Life Event Needs Assessments: Two Models for Measuring Preventable Mental Health Problems

Alex Zautra
Irwin Sandler

ABSTRACT. In this paper two complementary models are presented to guide needs assessment efforts for prevention programs. Each of these models focuses on events as the core elements in the study of human needs. One model is concerned with the nature and impact of stressful events on psychological distress; the other model is concerned with personal growth and development that may arise through integration of positive life experiences. After the models are described, suggestions are provided on how best to use them when conducting a prevention oriented needs assessment.

There are two major errors in how we typically conceptualize needs, particularly mental health needs. First we think people should not have them. Because of that, we blame those who do, referring to them as impaired, disturbed, etc. In a more enlightened but similarly flawed view, we blame the environments in which the needy live for contributing to their distress. The second error we make is thinking of needs solely as states of deprivation. When the person stops vocalizing discontent, we stop attending. In this process, we neglect self development needs.

Such errors have led several prevention theorists to criticize the conceptualization of needs as individual states of pathology. In objecting to the pathology model, they have proposed that distinctions be made both in the ends and means of prevention activities. Two

Requests for reprints should be addressed to Alex Zautra, Department of Psychology, Arizona State University, Tempe, AZ 85287.

35

such distinctions are most prominent: prevention of pathology versus the enhancement of well-being, and an individual focus versus a social environment focus.

Concern with reducing the incidence of different forms of pathology in the population is basic to traditional public health prevention. Within that framework scientific inquiry proceeds from identification of a disease of concern, study of how the rates of the disease are distributed in the population, construction of a theoretical model of the links in the chain of causation leading to the disorder, and development of prevention strategies designed to break the causal chain (Bloom, 1979). Bloom (1979) indicates, however, that recent psychiatric theory increasingly focuses on proximal (temporally recent) causes of disorder, particularly stressful life experiences. A particularly interesting feature of this model is that stress is not related to the etiology of a specific unique disorder; rather, it is seen as creating a vulnerability to a wide range of disorders.

Recently, strong dissatisfaction has been expressed with the goal of pathology prevention in favor of enhancement, empowerment, and the promotion of positive development. Several meanings can be discerned in people's concepts of positive development. Cowen (1977) proposes competence development as a strategy toward preventing the onset of disorder. "The view assumes that people are vulnerable to maladjustment when they lack specific skills needed to resolve personal problems" (p. 11). Rappaport (1981) on the other hand argues for empowerment rather than pathology prevention. Empowerment seeks to enhance people's ability to control their own lives as *an end in itself,* rather than as a means toward preventing pathology. Danish and D'Augelli (1980) similarly propose enhancement of human development as a preferable goal to prevention of pathology.

While these distinctions are conceptually meaningful, a point we will expand on later, they should not mask a focus which is shared across these frameworks. This common concern is with the experiences people have in their current life situations and on understanding the positive and negative impact of these experiences. Bloom (1979), for example, approaches these experiences from a stress theoretical base and is interested in their effects on increasing vulnerability to disease. Danish and D'Augelli (1980) see significant life events as markers of the course of development. One implication of this common focus is that the data base for planning both prevention and enhancement programs needs to include an assessment of the occurrence and effects of recent life experience.

A second distinction which is often drawn by prevention theorists is between focusing on social environments versus focusing on individuals (Cowen, 1977, 1980; Price, 1974). Price (1974), for example, describes system approaches to prevention as focusing on the effects of "key social institutions and settings in the environment which are presumed to affect human functioning for better or worse" (p. 292). The research agenda for the development of systems centered prevention approaches includes assessing the characteristics and effects of high impact social environments (e.g., schools, work places). Individual focused prevention, in contrast, proceeds by identifying people at risk and strengthening them to help ward off the disorder. Clearly, the assessment of the needs for prevention or enhancement planning should include both person and situational factors. Neither individual differences nor systemic forces can be ignored in understanding human needs.

To integrate these diverse approaches, we advocate a strategy for identifying prevention needs based on the assessment of person-environment transactions. The organizing element in this approach is the life event. Major events, such as marriage, divorce, and retirement, are used as discrete markers of a person's transactions with his/her environment. Relatively more minor events such as a negative social encounter, or a pleasing one, change the scale of assessment to daily transactions, but are also significant indicators of need (Kanner, Coyne, Schaefer, & Lazarus, 1981) in the patterns of everyday life. Both major life events and those that mark the quality of everyday life emerge from the natural fabric of a person's transactions within his/her environment.

Two Models of Need

In order to account for the full range of human needs we have developed two complementary models of how events impact psychological well being. These models are shown in Figures 1a and 1b. A Psychological Distress model is presented as a conceptual guide to needs assessment efforts focused on prevention of psychiatric symptomatology. The second model parallels the first in structure but has a different purpose. Called the Psychological Growth model, it identifies the steps by which a person may be said to enhance their personal development.

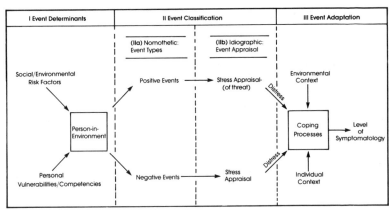

PSYCHOLOGICAL DISTRESS MODEL
FIGURE 1a

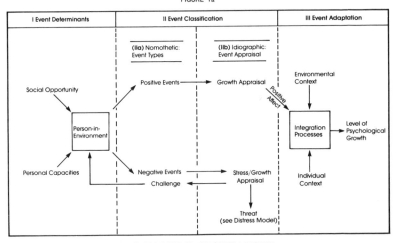

PSYCHOLOGICAL GROWTH MODEL
FIGURE 1b

FIGURES 1a & 1b. Two models related life events to mental health needs.

These models are drawn separately to correct the errors of the past in which personal growth needs, if they were dealt with at all, were treated either as residuals or made to depend upon successful adjustment to life stressors (e.g., Dohrenwend & Dohrenwend, 1980). The psychological processes underlying the two outcomes, the prevention of distress and optimization of functioning, are vastly different (Herzberg, 1966; Sanford, 1972); keeping the models separate helps preserve those differences.

Underlying the Psychological Distress model is the basic need to reduce and/or cope with harmful or otherwise threatening events that might result from person-environment transactions. Defense is the primary orientation. Understandably, a person finds no lasting gratification in these types of engagements with life. When the pressure is off and the stresses relaxed, the person stops defending. To continue to do so in the absence of threat is, after all, pathological.

Underlying growth-related activities is a very different orientation toward events. This orientation has been referred to as a need for competency (Cowen, 1977), effectance (White, 1959), intrinsic motivation (Deci, 1975), and personal growth (Herzberg, 1966). In its simplest form, satisfaction of this need provides what Nuttin (1973) has called "causality pleasure." As White (1959) and Herzberg (1966) have pointed out, this set of needs does not become stronger with deprivation; rather, it grows the more it is satisfied. Like a muscle, need for personal development is strengthened from use.

The process underlying growth motivation may appear paradoxical at first glance to needs assessors; attention to such needs would seem only to accelerate them. However, increases in need for mastery mean greater individuation and self-reliance and less, not more, dependence on community resources. Further, a person gives back to the environment by shaping, organizing, and creating new images from the supplies he/she receives. This is, after all, the psychological basis for cultural development.

Although they differ fundamentally on motivational grounds, the models are drawn together to highlight their many shared structural features. Both models posit person and environment factors that shape a "person-in-environment" nexus, which (see Figures 1a and 1b) in the model represents the condition of the person's relationship to his/her environment. Both models present two stages of Event Classification, through which experiences take on psychological significance. Both follow events through adaptation processes. Although they are different in the two models, they are the same in that adaptation is thought to rely on both environmental and individual contexts.

In essence, the models are used as devices to indicate what types of variables to include in a prevention needs assessment, and how such variables interrelate. Two models (Figures 1a, 1b) are explained step by step in the accompanying narrative beginning with the Event Determinants for the Psychological Distress model and ending with a discussion of Event Adaptation processes responsible for the integration of positive events that lead to growth.

PSYCHOLOGICAL DISTRESS MODEL

Event Determinants

In the distress model, the occurrence of events is seen as a consequence of both individual vulnerabilities and social/environmental risk factors. Individual characteristics which influence the probability of stressful events include personal traits, abilities, motivations, and the history of person-environment transactions. The conceptual point is that individuals are seen as active agents who initiate transactions with their environment. For example, people with a "Type A" personality, in their active quest to achieve, may, in fact, bring about the occurrence of *both* more positive and more negative events (Cresswell, Note 1). Roskies (1980) points out that Type As may interpret their attainments as being due to their life style, thus making it difficult for them to change their behavior and avoid future stressors.

Social environmental conditions can also effect the probability of the occurrence of events. For example, Myers, Lindenthal, and Pepper (1974) report that individuals of low social class experience an excess of high impact negative events. One can conceptualize many of the traditionally identified high risk situations (poverty, family conflict, parental mental illness) as situations in which there is a high frequency of stressful events. Illustratively, Kurdek (1981) has noted that the effects of divorce on children may be related to the stressors which occur in the post-divorce environment. Thus, the characteristics of the person and the situation in which they reside create the "person-in-environment" conditions shown in Figure 1a which determine the occurrence of life events.

Event Classification

The issue of identifying stressful life events is conceptually akin to identifying the critical stressful property of situations. This issue has been approached from a nomothetic and an idiographic perspective: *both* perspectives have value for needs assessment research.

The nomothetic approach assumes a commonality in the effects of events across people and identifies the stressful element of events on the basis of consensual judgment. Thus, the event characteristics are determined independent of the person's response to the event, which provides for a cleaner, less confounded measurement of the stimulus properties of those events that are stressful for a community group. Dohrenwend and Dohrenwend (1981) advocate this approach, and state that the stressfulness of events is based on culturally determined, normative beliefs about the meanings of events. Historically, the earliest identified stressful property of events was the amount of change and readjustment required by an event occurrence (Holmes & Masuda, 1974). A considerable body of evidence indicates that people can reliably rate the degree of change and readjustment (e.g., Kamaroff, Masuda, & Holmes, 1978). A competing model suggests that the aversiveness of the event rather than the degree of change is its critical stress property. Ross and Mirowsky (1979), for example, found that a measure based on simply adding the number of undesirable (i.e., aversive) events was a better predictor of psychological symptomatology than life event change measures.

In our distress model of life events, the positive versus negative distinction is made since this is the one most clearly distinguished in the literature. Some experiences may have both positive and negative features. In our models these features are treated as separate, albeit related, events. Other event characteristics have been identified [e.g., loss, entrance (Paykel, 1974), controllability (Dohrenwend & Martin, 1979)] and may be important for particular populations. Multivariate scaling techniques may be useful to identify event characteristics perceived as stressful by specific populations (Redfield & Stone, 1979; Sandler & Ramsay, 1980). For example, Sandler and Ramsay (1980) used factor analysis of event similarity ratings to identify dimensions clinicians used to conceptualize children's life events. Two dimensions (labelled as family troubles and entrance) related to both teacher and parent ratings of child adjustment problems.

In an idiographic approach, a stressful event is defined as a consequence of how an individual appraises an event. This approach is closer to how people actually experience an event. While it blurs the distinction between the event itself and the person's response, it provides a more accurate account of the degree of distress aroused by the event. In one illustrative approach, McGrath (1970) defines stress as the perception of an imbalance between environmental demands (such as work pressures) and individual ability to meet those demands. Lazarus and Launier (1978) suggest that it is the perception of harm, loss, and/or threat that leads to a stress response. Additionally, one might expect other event perceptions such as control (Glass & Singer, 1971), ego threat (Brown, 1974), and characterological self-blame (Janoff-Bulman, 1979) to affect their impact. Such perceptions may be a function of individual motivations, or past history, or even culturally prescribed themes (e.g., "machismo").

The distinction between idiographic and nomothetic approaches to defining stressful events provides an important resolution of the controversial issue of whether positive events are stressful (Gersten, Langner, Eisenberg, & Orzeck, 1974; Zautra & Reich, in press). There is little evidence that nomothetically defined positive events per se are stressful. These events are a mixed bag of anticipated events, some of which a person helped make happen. Few are truly unexpected major changes that require much adaptation. Positive events can idiographically be seen as threatening (e.g., "can I succeed at my new job"). As shown in Figure 1a, it is this perception of threat which can lead to distress.

Event Adaptation

Environmental context. As drawn in Figure 1a, both the environmental context in which events occur and the individual context affect coping processes. The environmental context includes social supports, which assist coping, and other significant experiences which may be occurring simultaneous to those of central concern. Several conceptually distinct measures of support are of interest, including who provides support, the content of the support provided, and how it is evaluated by the individual. Social network variables (e.g., size of network, dimensionality, multiplexity) are used to identify the sources of support (Mitchell & Trickett, 1980). There is some evidence that differential patterns of social connections lead to better adaptation in some situations than in others (Hirsch, 1980). Barrera (1981) identified six different types of social support: cognitive guidance, emotional support, positive feedback, social participation, task assistance, and advice and information. It is probable that each of these support functions will be most useful for different kinds of stressors.

Also, it is expected that experiencing stress in one life domain (e.g., family) makes an individual more vulnerable to the effects of stressors in a different area (e.g., job). Vossel and Froehlich (1979) found empirical support for this position in a study which demonstrated that the occurrence of negative non-job related life events increased feelings of job tension and reduced perceived task effectiveness. Other studies indicate that the occurrence of positive events reduces the stressful effect of negative events (Reich & Zautra, 1981; Cohen & McKay, in press).

Individual context. The individual context includes personal coping style, developmental life stage, and history of experiences with the same or similar stressors. Several personality characteristics have been identified which affect the stressful impact of events, including locus of control (Johnson & Sarason, 1978; Sandler & Lakey, 1982), hardiness (Kobasa, 1979), and Type A personality (Glass, 1977). While there is evidence that some coping characteristics buffer the effects of a wide range of stressors, it may also be that some ways of coping may be useful for meeting some stress demands but not others. Katz, Weiner, Gallagher, and Hellman (1970) report that while denial was helpful in regulating the emotions of breast cancer biopsy patients, it also led some patients to delay seeking treatment when perceiving early symptoms.

Developmental tasks play an important role in how people cope with significant events. Danish and D'Augelli (1980) point out that events can be seen as markers of the course of adult development. There are normative times for events to occur and "off-times" when events are developmentally atypical. For developmentally normative events (e.g., having a child, retiring), their meaning can be more readily understood in terms of the developmentally salient issues (e.g., Levinson, 1978) when they occur "on-time." There are also more likely to be social support resources readily available to aid coping. In support of this proposition, Goodhart and Zautra (in press) found that elderly residents with more negative "off-time" events reported greater psychological distress and a lower quality of life.

Distress Outcomes

Finally, the possible distressful effects of events need to be considered. Traditionally, these have been studied as negative mood, psychological symptomatology, physical illness, and poorer work and academic effectiveness. A review of these is beyond the scope of this paper (see Dohrenwend, Shrout, Egri, & Mendelsohn, 1980; Link & Dohrenwend, 1982).

One important set of outcomes often overlooked by researchers is how a stressful event can influence the occurrence of other negative events. Cues of such outcomes would show up first in event-event correlations. Inspection of those relationships for different community groups can sometimes be the first concrete sign of significant differences in how members of different groups adapt to events. Since few investigators have displayed such analyses, we provide one below as an illustration.

In Table 1, correlations are given between the life event "End of a love relationship" and other stressful life events across four subgroups of a representative sample of 498 community residents (see Zautra et al., 1982, for a description of the sample). Basic group

Table 1

Negative Event Correlates of End of Love Relationship

for Four Community Groups

Events	Men & Women Age 18-24 (N=118)	Men Age 25-54 (N=110)	Women Age 25-56 (N=145)	Men & Women Age 55+ (N=125)	Total Sample (N=498)
Major Marital Conflict	.59	.53	.56	.50	.56
Sexual Difficulties	-	.26	-	-	.11
Death of Spouse	-	-	-	.28	-
Death of Family Member	-	-	-	.33	-
Death of Close Friend	.28	-	-	-	-
Trouble with Boss	.25	-	-	-	.19
Psychological Problems	.30	-	.32	.21	.25
Personal Injury	.28	-	-	-	-
Decrease in Social Activity	-	-	.26	-	-
Major Personal Embarrassment	-	-	.20	.22	.11
Increased Boredom	-	-	.24	-	-
Personal Frustration	-	-	.31	-	.21
More Arguments	-	-	.26	.30	.14
Worse Finances	-	-	.30	-	.14
Less Sleep	-	-	.21	-	.13
Child Illness	-	-	.24	-	-
Child has Social Problem	-	-	.27	-	-
Begin New Relationship	-	.31	.46	.38	.32

Note: Only statistically significant correlations ($p < .05$) are shown in this table. All non-significant correlations are represented by a dash.

differences had already been uncovered on how events were related to psychological distress, justifying a closer look at these event-event relationships. In those prior analyses, correlations between negative events and distress were .05 for married men between the ages of 25 and 54 ($n = 77$), and .38 for unmarried men of the same age ($n = 33$). The correlations were significantly higher both for married women, $r(42) = .48$, and unmarried women, $r(18) = .64$, of the same age as the men.

What is most apparent from Table 1, are the large differences in event-event relationships between men and women in the mid-age ranges. End of a love relationship brought along with it a set of complex problems for women including less social activity, worsening finances, and more problems among the children. Their problems appeared to multiply. For men, end of a love relationship brought only a small increase in the probability of sexual difficulties. While the beginning of a new relationship appears more probable for women than men here, a separate analysis showed that men were quicker to report a new relationship along with the event "marital troubles" than women. Apparently, new relationships began soon after (and may have caused) marital troubles for men. Although causal linkages are not possible to confirm from data like these, they do provide a base for supporting hypotheses about such causes. The findings lead directly to the identification of high risk groups and provide concrete evidence of the nature of the difficulties they face as a result of stressful life events.

PERSONAL GROWTH AND DEVELOPMENT MODEL

Event Determinants

In this growth model, shown in Figure 1b, evidence of personal development begins with the assessment of events that signify either successful transactions with the environment or opportunities for success. Both a personal history of growth experiences and social opportunities shape a matrix of personal involvements with the environment that lead to positive events. For example, community residents with higher education have been shown to report a greater number of satisfying events (Goodstein, Zautra, & Goodhart, 1982). Enriched jobs have led employees to rate up the number of their satisfying work experiences (Herzberg & Zautra, 1976), and growth oriented organizational climates (Moos & Moos, in press) may encourage activities leading to mastery experiences.

In passing, however, it is important to note that not all desirable events, even when they involve personal mastery, are good for the community. Criminal activity, when successful, can lead to greater self-worth, even though it is quite destructive to others. Such activities may be the best career available in some subcultures. It is interesting how frequently such behavior is misunderstood as a response to stress. In doing so, Figure 1a is used rather than 1b, which leads to the mistaken conclusion that the removal of stressors or better coping skills will automatically lead to diminished criminal activity.

Event Classification

Both nomothetic and idiographic classification aid in identifying whether an event is growth enhancing. The most straightforward classification is based on an event's desirability. When items from event inventories are written unambiguously to show the direction of the change, consensus ratings may yield high agreement on the social value of the event. For example, although an event such as "change in job responsibilities" would not be reliably rated by observers, the event "increase in job responsibility" would likely be rated as socially desirable by a high proportion of judges (Zautra, Kochanowicz, & Goodhart, 1982).

Herzberg (1966) and others (e.g., Deci, 1975) have argued that not all positive events lead to psychological growth and personal development. Other qualities of events, such as the degree of mastery, personal involvement, and internal causation underlying events, are thought to play an important role. Zautra and Reich (1980) distinguished between origin and pawn events based on consensual ratings of the degree of personal causality implicit in the occurrence of the events. Origin events, those a person intended and helped make happen, led to a higher quality of life overall in that study than did positive pawn events; those that occurred out of a person's control.

Subjective appraisals are especially important in the study of benefits obtained from events. The degree of positive affect associated with an event depends greatly upon how a person appraises its contribution to his/her own plans and interests. The alternative was already noted in the distress model; positive events can be seen as threatening current plans, leading potentially to distress.

A number of researchers have pointed out ways that cognitive processes affect appraisals of events. While investigators differ in their choice of cognitive dimensions (e.g., Abramson, Seligman & Teasdale, 1978; Gong-Guy & Hammen, 1980; Weiner, 1979), there is evidence that internal attributions and perceptions of control influence whether a person shows gain or loss in well-being as a function of events (Weiner, 1979). There also are reciprocal influences between positive event types and perceptions of control that should not go unnoticed. Positive events, per se, appear to boost feelings of control. Winners of games of chance have been shown to display more confidence in their capacity to control future chance outcomes than losers (Langer, 1977). Untested in such laboratory studies, however, is whether expectations which are built on chance events lead to "false hope" (Murrell & Norris, Note 2) and eventual disappointment. Zautra and Reich (1980) found, for example, that pawn events actually coincided with subsequent reports of greater negative affect.

A negative event may stimulate personal growth activity depending upon whether it is appraised as a challenge or a threat (Lazarus et al., 1980). Figure 1b shows this relationship. This relationship is drawn to reflect the fact that few events are actually transformed from negative to positive, growth enhancing experiences through appraisal processes alone. In the model (see Figure 1b), an event appraised as a challenge becomes a new input in the person-environment relationship. The outcome of that perceived challenge depends on many additional factors. It itself should be counted as an event. Research is fairly consistent with this aspect of the model. Investigators have had little success finding measures that show any "silver lining" from negative life events (e.g., Goodhart, Note 3). At best, researchers have suggested constructs such as hardiness (Kobasa, 1979) and coping style (Folkman & Lazarus, 1980) that appear to lessen the harm of life stressors. Enhancement of functioning has not been demonstrated, and may reflect only wishful thinking on the part of investigators and the victims of stressors outside of their control.

The failure to find positive benefits from negative experiences may be due to the use of major crisis events rather than less overwhelming events such as those assessed in daily event inventories.

Bandura (1982) has shown that breaking up insurmountable tasks into smaller steps can aid the development of self-efficacy. The key may be whether the person perceives that his/her efforts can change the outcome (Lazarus et al., 1980; Weiner, 1979). In such cases as well, challenge felt must be put to work in a person's interaction with their environment, as the model shows.

Event Adaptation: Integration Processes

The process of integration is a key to long term personal growth benefit from events (Jahoda, 1958). Integration depends upon how the event fits with deeper structures, both within the person and in the person's relationship to his/her environment.

Individual context. We have already alluded to how individual differences in plans and interests help determine whether an event reinforces personal development. Further, whether a mastery experience is successfully integrated within a person's system of beliefs about him/herself depends also on the conditions of that system (Valliant, 1977). Epstein (1979) has perhaps the most fully articulated model of how events interact with the self-system, a personal set of theoretical constructs that define who they are in relation to their social environment. According to Epstein (1979), events can confirm and extend the self theory; they can also fail to support or even challenge it. Considerable information can be obtained about how likely an event will lead to growth by determining how well experiences fit with interests and needs. The pattern of responses to events may also reveal individual differences in cognitive style and openness to growth. Herzberg (1966), for example, has identified groups who fail to develop psychologically from experiences because they view positive events as useful only for reducing dissatisfaction, and not valuable for their own sake.

Environmental context. The structure and climate of social exchange can also facilitate or actively interfere with integration of mastery experiences (Moos & Moos, 1983). External rewards have been shown to undermine or otherwise reduce intrinsic motivation (see Condry, 1977, for a review). Such rewards are thought to influence the motivational context surrounding performance, shifting perceptions from an internal to an external locus of causation. Not all rewards undermine performance, however; some have cue value signifying to the person that his/her efforts were of sufficient quality. Along these lines, verbal praise has been shown to strengthen interest in some tasks (e.g., Deci, 1975).

We suggest that the analysis of event-event correlations would be useful to gauge specific person-environment responses to positive experiences. Some social systems may be structured such that negative experiences accompany positive ones. Spouses in a competitive family may anger one another with their successes, for example. Rites of passage (ritualistic but nevertheless painful negative events) often accompany developmental changes. Furthermore, different groups may be differentially affected. Kanner et al. (1981) found that daily uplifts were more highly correlated with hassles for women than men. Methods of analysis are still in an undeveloped stage and care would need to be taken to differentiate those events that clearly were due to responses of the social environment from those that arise from personal action. Nonetheless, the way events are linked together in a person's life provide rich data on the nature of transactions between persons and their environments, and how easily a valued event is integrated within a person's system of relations with their environment.

Growth Outcomes

Personal development is measurable, at least in part, by the outcomes of satisfying events themselves. Positive affects associated with events (e.g., Bradburn, 1969) are signals that the events are occurring which are congruent with a person's interests and plans (Westbrook, 1976). They are, for the most part, only trace measures of personal development, however. Life satisfaction indices (e.g., Andrews & Withey, 1976; Cantril, 1969) provide more stable measures of perceived success in major transactions with the environment.

Another approach has been to rely on measures of generalized beliefs in self-efficacy (e.g., Gurin & Gurin, 1976), self reliance (Pearlin & Schooler, 1982), and positive mental health (Wright, 1971). For the elderly, Lawton, Moss, Fulcomer, & Kleban (1981) have developed subscales to assess perceived competency in tasks of daily living, and Paul and his colleagues (Note 4) have developed a competency instrument for college students. While these measures are also related to successful adjustment to stressful events, they have the advantage of providing an overall criterion which is a face valid measure of attitudes about the self.

TRANSLATING MODELS INTO PRACTICE:
LIFE EVENT NEEDS ASSESSMENT

The models we present are only rough blueprints for assessing needs. They are based on our review of recent theory and supporting empirical literature on how events affect psychological well-being. Still, the bricks and mortar are missing. We wish to extend our treatment of these issues to provide some guidance to the investigator wishing to apply these models to perform a prevention oriented needs assessment survey of community groups.

First, knowledge of the community is important in any assessment. This is true whatever model is employed. Needs assessment research necessarily applies theoretical models of growth and/or symptomatology to specific settings. A familiarity with the culture and history of the setting is critical in making the translation from general models to specific needs. A number of techniques have been used successfully in community settings to identify public perceptions of social problems including surveys of key informants and community forums (Warheit, Bell, & Schwab, 1975). Archival data is often available on the geographic distribution of selected demographic groups. Service use data is also generally available though often of questionable reliability.

Second, the research focus should be clearly defined. Most investigators will have already selected the class of problems within which they plan to work (e.g., mental health, criminal justice, alcoholism). They need to determine which one of the two models we presented best fits their underlying premises about the nature of prevention needs and is consistent with the level and depth of prevention programming that they have the resources to develop. Each model provides a number of points of intervention, ranging from the identification of social forces responsible for the increased frequency of stressful life events to the study of individual coping effectiveness. While data on aspects of each full model would be useful, the particular focus of the investigator should receive the most thorough assessment. Thus, for example, if the investigator has a particular interest in the development and enhancement of social support, it would be important to obtain a multi-method assessment of this construct (e.g., social networks, support functions, supportive behaviors received; Sandler & Barrera, Note 5). Further, for any social problem, there are a wide range of targets: individuals, families, organizations, and the community itself. The data should be collected and aggregated to match the ecological level of planned interventions. For example, studies of families should use families (not individual family members) as the units of analysis.

Third, construction of a valid event list is necessary. A representative list of significant life events for the population under study is crucial to this kind of needs assessment. Tailor-made life event lists have been developed for several populations including college students (Sandler & Lakey, 1982; Levine & Perkins, Note 6), community college students (Bauman, Sandler, & Braver, Note 7), and New York City residents (Dohrenwend et al., 1978). Several steps are useful in generating a representative list of significant events. A critical incident technique can be employed either in an interview or questionnaire to have community residents and key informants from the community identify significant events. Sandler (see Sandler & Lakey, 1982), for example, asked over 200 college students to identify all events whose occurrence had a significant impact on them, generating 1500 events. This list was paired down by combining similar items to comprise a college student event list of 111 items. Attempts have also been made to develop lists of positive life events (Flanagan, 1978; Herzberg, 1966; Zautra, Kochanowicz, & Goodhart, 1982).

Recent research has also focused on assessing the more routine events in everyday life (Epstein, 1976; MacPhillamy & Lewinsohn, 1982; Moss & Lawton, 1982; Kanner et al., 1982; Reich & Zautra, 1983). Using time budget survey methods, Robinson (1983) and Moss and Lawton (1982) have coded daily activities as either obligatory or discretionary. Lewinsohn and his colleagues (see MacPhillamy & Lewinsohn, 1982) have identified pleasant and unpleasant events and related them to depressed mood and affect. Kanner et al. (1981) have labelled events as either "hassles" or "uplifts," finding them superior to life events in predicting psychological well-being. Reich and Zautra (1983) have developed methods of studying two kinds of events, "demands" and "desires." A balance of coping successfully with demands and finding time to meet desires is expected to lead to heightened life satisfaction. Provided the assessment of daily events is ecologically valid, this approach provides greater specificity compared to major event assessments on how people find satisfaction and distress in their lives.

Fourth, testable hypotheses should be stated. The value of making a priori predictions is that there is more power to identify relationships and to have confidence in their replicability. There is an almost endless number of correlation coefficients to compute between events and outcomes in a survey study. By establishing hypotheses, the investigator orders the analysis in a way that is most consistent with his/her assumptions and theory. The theory may be based either on prior research on stress and coping or on specific observations about the particular setting or population of interest. Further, findings contrary to expectations, when they occur, can have a strong influence on our way of thinking about the community and its needs. Learning from one's own misperceptions does not take place, however, unless the person states clearly what he/she expects.

We leave out attention to the design of surveys and data collection procedures which normally would be discussed at this point. Those problems are dealt with much more thoroughly elsewhere than is possible here (see Bradburn & Sudman, 1980; Sudman, 1976; Survey Research Center, 1976; also for a discussion of the use of path models and cross-lagged panel designs see Cook & Campbell, 1979). There are no unique procedural problems posed by the models presented here.

Finally, the analysis of event data should proceed in logical order, broken into several distinct steps to address central questions in a prevention oriented needs assessment. In Table 2 we outline these steps. They correspond to major stages presented in the models shown in Figure 1a, b.

I.   What are the determinants of events? Both social environment and individual difference variables can be used to predict the frequency of occurrence of significant events. For example, in a survey study of older community residents one might be interested in whether neighborhood characteristics predict the occurrence of positive events. At an individual level one might focus on income or education as event predictors.

IIa. What kinds of events are associated with distress and/or growth outcomes? Events can be grouped into meaningful subsets based either on theory or pilot observation of the community. Such subsets can be used as separate variables to predict criteria of interest (e.g., life satisfaction or symptomatology). Illustratively, Sandler & Ramsay (1980) found that family troubles and entrance events, but not loss or sibling problem events, accounted for the adjustment problems of inner-city children.

Table 2

Illustrative Data Analysis for Life Events Based Needs Assessment

Needs Assessment Questions	Distress Model: Variables	Growth Model: Variables	Implications for Prevention Programming
I What are the determinants of event occurrence?	Setting hazards, social risk factors Individual pathology	Opportunities Individual talents	Intervention to reduce occurrence of negative events and increase occurrence of positive events for identified groups Intervention to help people anticipate events
IIA What kinds of events are stressful and/or growth enhancing?	Loss events, family troubles	Positive and mastery events	Focused intervention on specific sub-sets of events
IIB How are these events appraised?	Degree of harm/loss, threat, uncontrollability	Degree of personal causation, how event fits with plans and interests	Community education/workshops and action to change event appraisals
IIIA What social environment variables moderate the effects of events on outcomes?	Social support, other positive and negative events	Organizational climate, other events	Strengthen the development of support networks Organizational intervention to improve management practices
IIIB What individual differences moderate effects of events on outcomes?	Hardiness, stable coping styles	Cognitive style, personality structure	Improve coping skills of identified individuals. Reduce negative event fallout from positive experiences

53

IIb. How are the events appraised? The subjective appraisal of events by respondents provides unique information which might help to explain the differential effects of events across groups. For example, do some groups make more ability attributions for negative events and fewer individual competence attributions for positive events?

III. What variables (individual and social environment) moderate the effects of events on outcomes? Here hypotheses made about factors which moderate the relationship between events and outcomes are empirically tested. The stress buffering role of social support (Heller & Swindle, 1981; Cohen & McKay, 1982), and the immunity to stress of the hardy personality (Kobasa, 1979) are two such hypotheses.

SUMMARY

We have attempted to sketch out a transactional approach to prevention oriented needs assessment. The two measurement models we described represent our synthesis of current theory and empirical evidence of the determinants of distress and psychological growth. While others have attempted to place both distress and growth components of well-being in the same model (e.g., Dohrenwend & Dohrenwend, 1981), we have found it more consistent with the evidence to define the two as separate processes. By translating some of the model components, we wish to encourage the application of life event oriented needs assessment, a method which should provide concrete evidence of psychological troubles and growth opportunities about to happen in community life.

REFERENCE NOTES

1. Cresswell, D. *Type A behavior pattern, negative life events, and symptomatology.* Unpublished Doctoral Dissertation, Arizona State University, 1981.

2. Murrell, S.A., & Norris, F.H. *Resources, life events and changes in psychological states: A conceptual framework.* Unpublished paper. University of Louisville, Urban Studies Center, Louisville, Kentucky 40292.

3. Goodhart, D. *Cognitive resolution of ordinary life crises and psychological well-being.* Doctoral dissertation, Arizona State University, August 1980.

4. Paul, S. (Chairman). *Prelude to prevention: Personal competencies, social networks and adjustment.* Symposium presented at the meeting of the American Psychological Association, Washington, D.C., August 1982.

5. Sandler, I.N., & Barrera, M. *Social support as a stress buffer: A multi-method in-*

vestigation. Paper presented at the meeting of the American Psychological Association, Montreal, September 1980.

6. Levine, M., & Perkins, D.V. *Tailor made life events scales.* Paper presented at the meeting of the American Psychological Association, Montreal, 1980.

7. Bauman, D., Sandler, I.N., & Braver, S. *Using a tailor made life event scale for needs assessment research.* Paper presented at the meeting of the American Psychological Association, Washington, D.C., August 1982.

REFERENCES

Bandura, A. Self-efficacy mechanism in human agency. *American Psychologist,* 1982, *37,* 122-147.

Barrera, M. Social support in the adjustment of pregnant adolescents: Assessment issues. In B.H. Gottlieb (Ed.), *Social networks and social support.* Beverly Hills: Sage, 1981.

Barrera, M., & Ainley, S.L. The structure of social support: A conceptual and empirical analysis. *Journal of Community Psychology,* 1983, in press.

Bloom, B.L. Prevention of mental disorders: Recent advances in theory and practice. *Community Mental Health Journal,* 1979, *15,* 179-191.

Bradburn, N. *The structure of psychological well-being.* Chicago: Aldine, 1969.

Bradburn, N., & Sudman, S. *Improving interview method and questionnaire design.* San Francisco: Jossey-Bass, 1980.

Bulman, R.J. Characterological versus behavioral self-blame: Inquiries into depression and rape. *Journal of Personality and Social Psychology,* 1979, *37,* 1798-1809.

Cohen, S., & McKay, G. Social support, stress and the buffering hypothesis: An empirical review. In A. Baum, J.E. Singer, & S.E. Taylor (Eds.), *Handbook of psychology and health* (Vol. 4). Hillsdale, N.J.: Erlbaum, 1982.

Condry, J. Enemies of exploration: Self-initiated versus other initiated learning. *Journal of Personality and Social Psychology,* 1971, *35,* 459-477.

Cook, T.D., & Campbell, D.T. *Quasi-experimentation: Design & analyses issues for field studies.* Chicago: Rand McNally, 1979.

Cowen, E.L. Baby-steps toward primary prevention. *American Journal of Community Psychology,* 1977, *5,* 481-491.

Cowen, E.L. The wooing of primary prevention. *American Journal of Community Psychology,* 1980, *8,* 258-284.

Danish, S.J., & D'Augelli, A.R. Promoting competence and enhancing development through life development intervention. In L.A. Bond & J.C. Rosen (Eds.), *Primary prevention of psychopathology* (Vol. 4). Hanover, N.H.: University Press of New England, 1980.

Deci, E.L. *Intrinsic Motivation.* New York: Plenum Press, 1975.

Dohrenwend, B.S., & Dohrenwend, B.P. What is a stressful life event. In L.H. Selye (Ed.), *Selye's guide to stress research* (Vol. 1). New York: Van Nostrand Reinhold, 1980.

Dohrenwend, B.P., Shrout, P.E., Egri, G., & Mendelsohn, E.S. Nonspecific. Psychological distress and other dimensions of psychopathology. *Archives of General Psychiatry,* 1980, *37,* 1229-1236.

Dohrenwend, B.S., Krasnsoff, L., Askenasy, A.R., & Dohrenwend, B.P. Exemplification of a method for scaling life events: The PERI life events scale. *Journal of Health and Social Behavior,* 1978, *19,* 205-229.

Epstein, S. Anxiety, arousal and the self-concept. In I.G. Sarason & C.D. Spielberger (Eds.), *Stress and anxiety* (Vol. 3). Washington, D.C.: Hemisphere, 1976.

Epstein, S. The stability of behavior I: On predicting most of the people much of the time. *Journal of Personality and Social Psychology,* 1979, *37,* 1097-1126.

Flanagan, J.C. A research approach to improving our quality of life. *American Psychologist,* 1978, *33,* 138-147.

Folkman, S., & Lazarus, R. An analysis of coping in a middle-aged community sample. *Journal of Health and Social Behavior*, 1980, *21*, 219-239.

Glass, D.C. *Behavior patterns, stress, and coronary disease.* Hillsdale, N.J.: Erlbaum, 1977.

Glass, D.C., & Singer, J.E. *Urban stress: Experiments on noise and social stressors.* New York: Academic Press, 1972.

Gurin, G., & Gurin, P. Personal efficacy and the ideology of individual responsibility. In B. Strumpel (Ed.), *Economic means for human needs.* Ann Arbor: Institute for Social Research, 1976.

Gong-Guy, E., & Hammen, C. Causal perceptions of stressful events in depressed and nondepressed out patients. *Journal of Abnormal Psychology*, 1980, *89*, 662-669.

Goodstein, J., Zautra, A., & Goodhart, D. A test of the utility of social indicators for behavioral health service planning. *Social Indicator Research*, 1982, *10*, 273-295.

Heller, K., & Swindle, R.W. Social networks, perceived social support and coping with stress. In R.D. Felner, L.A. Jason, J. Moritsugu, & S.S. Farber (Eds.), *Preventive psychology: Theory, research and practice in community intervention.* New York: Pergamon Press, 1982.

Hirsch, B.J. Natural support systems and coping with major life changes. *American Journal of Community Psychology*, 1980, *8*, 159-172.

Herzberg, F. *Work and the nature of man.* New York: Thomas Y. Crowell, 1966.

Herzberg, F., & Zautra, A. Orthodox job enrichment: Measuring true quality in job satisfaction. *Personnel*, 1976, *53*, 54-68.

Holmes, T.H., & Masuda, M. Life change and illness susceptibility. In B.S. Dohrenwend & B.P. Dohrenwend (Eds.), *Stressful life events: Their nature and effects.* New York: Wiley, 1974.

Hurst, M.W., Jenkins, C.D., & Rose, R.M. The assessment of life change stress: A comparative and methodological critique. *Psychosomatic Medicine*, 1978, *40*, 126-141.

Johnson, J.H., & Sarason, I.G. Moderator variables in life stress research. In I.G. Sarason & C.D. Spielberger (Eds.), *Stress and anxiety* (Vol. 6). Washington, D.C.: Hemisphere, 1979.

Kanner, A.D., Coyne, J.C., Schaefer, C., & Lazarus, R.S. Comparison of two modes of stress management: Daily hassles and uplifts versus major life events. *Journal of Behavioral Medicine*, 1981, *4*, 1-39.

Katz, J.L., Weiner, H., Gallagher, T.F., & Hellman, L. Stress, distress and ego defenses: Psychoendocrine responses to impending breast tumor biopsy. *Archives of General Psychiatry*, 1970, *23*, 131-142.

Kobasa, S.C. Stressful life events, personality and health: An inquiry into hardiness. *Journal of Personality and Social Psychology*, 1979, *37*, 1-11.

Komaroff, A.L., Masuda, M., & Holmes, T.H. The social readjustment rating scale: A comparative study of Negro, Mexican and White Americans. *Journal of Psychosomatic Research*, 1968, *12*, 156-163.

Kurdek, J.A. An integrative perspective on children's divorce adjustment. *American Psychologist*, 1981, *36*, 856-866.

Langer, E.J. The psychology of chance. *Journal for the Theory of Social Behavior*, 1977, *7*, 185-207.

Langner, T.S. A twenty-two item screening score of psychiatric symptoms indicating impairment. *Journal of Health and Human Behavior*, 1962, *3*, 269-275.

Lawton, M.P., Moss, M., Fulcomer, M., & Kleban, M.H. A research and service oriented multilevel assessment instrument. *Journal of Gerontology*, 1982, *37*, 91-99.

Lazarus, R.S., Kanner, A.D., & Folkman, S. Emotions: A cognitive-phenomenological analysis. In Plutchik, R. & H. Kellerman (Eds.), *Theories of emotion* (Vol. 1). New York: Academic Press, 1980.

Lazarus, R., & Launier, R. Stress-related transactions between person and environment. In L.A. Pervin & M. Lewis (Eds.), *Perspectives in interactional psychology.* New York: Plenum, 1978.

Levinson, D.J. *The seasons of a man's life.* New York: Knopf, 1978.

Link, B., & Dohrenwend, B.P. Formulation about hypotheses about the true prevalence of demoralization in the United States. In B.P. Dohrenwend, M.S. Gould, B. Link, R. Hewgebauer, & R. Wunsch-Hitzig (Eds.), *Mental illness in the United States.* New York: Praeger, 1980.

MacPhillamy, D.J., & Lewinsohn, P.M. The pleasant events schedule: Studies on reliability, validity and scale writer correlation. *Journal of Consulting and Clinical Psychology,* 1982, *50,* 363-380.

McGrath, J.E. A conceptual formulation for research on stress. In J.E. McGrath (Ed.), *Social and psychological factors in stress.* New York: Holt, 1970.

Mitchell, R.E., & Trickett, E.J. An analysis of the effects and determinants of social networks. *Community Mental Health Journal,* 1980, *16,* 27-44.

Moos, R., & Moos, B.S. Adaptation and the quality of life in work and family settings. *Journal of Community Psychology,* 1983.

Moss, M.S., & Lawton, M.P. Time budgets of older people: A window on four life styles. *Journal of Gerontology,* 1982, *37,* 115-123.

Myers, J.K., Lindenthal, J.J., & Pepper, M.P. Social class, life events, and psychiatric symptoms: A longitudinal study. In B.S. Dohrenwend & B.P. Dohrenwend (Eds.), *Stressful life events: Their nature and effects.* New York: Wiley, 1974.

Nuttin, J.R. Pleasure and reward in human motivation and learning. In D.E. Berlyne & K.B. Madsen (Eds.), *Pleasure, reward and preference.* New York: Academic Press, 1973.

Paykel, E.S. Life stress and psychiatric disorder: Applications of the clinical approach. In B.S. Dohrenwend & B.P. Dohrenwend (Eds.), *Stressful life events: Their nature and effects.* New York: Wiley, 1974.

Pearlin, L.I., Lieberman, M.A., Menaghan, E.G., & Mullan, J.T. The stress process. *Journal of Health and Social Behavior,* 1981, *22,* 337-356.

Price, R.H. Etiology, the social environment, and the prevention of psychological dysfunction. In P. Insel & R.H. Moos (Eds.), *Health and the social environment.* Lexington, Mass.: D.C. Heath, 1974.

Rappaport, J. In praise of paradox. *American Journal of Community Psychology,* 1981, *9,* 1-26.

Reich, J., & Zautra, A. Demands and desires in daily life: Some influences on well-being. *American Journal of Community Psychology,* 1983, *11,* 41-58.

Reich, J., & Zautra, A. Life events and personal causation: Some relationships with distress and satisfaction. *Journal of Personality and Social Psychology,* 1981, *41,* 1002-1012.

Roskies, E. Considerations in developing a treatment program for the coronary-prone (type A) behavior pattern. In P. Davidson & S. Davidson (Eds.), *Behavioral medicine: Changing health life styles.* New York: Brunner/Mazel, 1980.

Robinson, J.P. Environmental differences in how Americans use time: The case for subjective and objective indicators. *Journal of Community Psychology,* 1983.

Ross, C.E., & Mirowsky, J. A comparison of life-event-weighting schemes: Change, undesirability, and effect-proportional indices. *Journal of Health and Social Behavior,* 1979, *20,* 166-177.

Sandler, I.N., & Ramsay, T.B. Dimensional analysis of children's stressful life events. *American Journal of Community Psychology,* 1980, *8,* 285-302.

Sandler, I.N., & Lakey, B. Locus of control as a stress moderator: The role of control perceptions and social support. *American Journal of Community Psychology,* 1982, *10,* 65-80.

Sanford, N. Is the concept of prevention necessary or useful? In S.E. Golamn & C. Eisdorfer (Eds.), *Handbook of community mental health.* New York: Appleton-Century-Crofts, 1972.

Sudman, S. *Applied sampling.* New York: Academic Press, 1976.

Survey Research Center. *Interviewer's manual* (Rev. ed.). Ann Arbor: Institute for Social Research, 1976.

Valliant, G. *Adaptation to life.* Boston: Little, Brown, 1977.

Vossel, G., & Froehlich, W.D. Life stress, job tension, and subjective reports of task performance effectiveness: A cross-lagged correlations analysis. In J.G. Sarason & C.D. Spielberger (Eds.), *Stress and anxiety* (Vol. 6). New York: Hemisphere, 1979.

Warheit, G.J., Bell, R.A., & Schwab, J.J. *Planning for change: Needs assessment approaches.* Rockville, Maryland: Department of Health, Education and Welfare, 1975.

Weiner, B. A theory of motivation for some classroom experiences. *Journal of Educational Psychology,* 1979, *71,* 3-25.

Weinstein, N.D. Unrealistic optimism about future life events. *Journal of Personality and Social Psychology,* 1980, *59,* 806-826.

Westbrook. M.T. Positive affect: A method of content analysis for verbal samples. *Journal of Consulting and Clinical Psychology,* 1976, *44,* 715-719.

White, R.W. Motivation reconsidered: The concept of competence. *Psychological Review,* 1959, *66,* 297-333.

Wright, L. Components of positive mental health. *Journal of Consulting and Clinical Psychology,* 1971, *36,* 277-280.

Zautra, A., & Reich, J.W. Positive life events and reports of well-being: Some useful distinctions. *American Journal of Community Psychology,* 1980, *8,* 657-670.

Zautra, A., Kochanowicz, N., & Goodhart, D. Surveying of quality of life in the community. In R. Bell, M. Sundel, J. Aponte, & S. Murrel (Eds.), *Assessing health and human service needs: Concepts, methods and applications.* New York: Human Sciences Press, 1982.

Assessing Social Support as a Prevention Resource: An Illustrative Study

Manuel Barrera, Jr.
Pamela Balls

ABSTRACT. Social support is popularly regarded as a naturally existing resource that acts to prevent disorder by buffering the effects of stress or by meeting individuals' fundamental needs for meaningful human attachment. The present paper begins by discussing approaches to measuring social support that might be adopted in needs assessment research. A prospective study of 74 young mothers is described to illustrate the use of multiple measures of support in investigating their relationship to birth outcome measures. In this study, direct relationships were found between birth outcome indices and measures of both prenatal negative life events and psychological distress. Social support network size showed stress moderating effects when Apgar scores served as the outcome measure. When the presence of birth complications served as the criterion variable, moderating effects were also found for a support satisfaction measure. The paper closes by examining some implications of this study for needs assessments designed for the planning of preventive interventions.

The growing literature on social support has portrayed it as a concept that can valuably contribute to an understanding of how physical and psychological disorders can be prevented. Social sup-

Some of the research described in this paper was supported by a Faculty Grant-in-Aid that was awarded to the first author by Arizona State University. The second author was supported by a National Institute of Mental Health predoctoral training fellowship. Special appreciation is extended to Alfonso Bravo of the Arizona Department of Health Services, Carol Lamond-Walker of the Phoenix Union School District, Pat Baird of the Maricopa County Health Department, and their coworkers whose active cooperation made this study possible.

A version of this paper was presented at the annual meeting of the Western Psychological Association, Los Angeles, April 1981.

All correspondence should be sent to Manuel Barrera, Jr., Department of Psychology, Arizona State University, Tempe, AZ 85287.

59

port is thought to aid in the prevention of disorder through a number of possible mechanisms. As key community gatekeepers, social support network members are viewed as serving the secondary prevention functions of early detection and referral (Gottlieb & Hall, 1980; Gourash, 1978). Some have argued that there are basic human needs for affiliation and attachment and that when these needs are not met individuals are likely to experience psychological disorder and illness (Bowlby, 1969; Henderson, 1977; Weiss, 1969). From this perspective, social support serves a primary prevention function by satisfying fundamental needs for meaningful human attachment.

The preventive functions of social support have been discussed most prominently in the context of social support's role as a "buffer" or moderator of life stress. Reviews of the recent empirical research on this topic have noted a number of methodological and conceptual shortcomings, but overall the results appear to suggest that social support is an effective coping resource for assisting individuals in meeting the demands of stressful life experiences (Cohen & McKay, in press; Heller & Swindle, in press). Certainly the results have shown enough promise to warrant continued research on how social support might function to prevent forms of psychological distress and physical illness.

While research has been encouraging thus far, the clarification of several issues could further strengthen the contribution of social support to needs assessments that are designed for the planning of preventive interventions. One purpose of the present paper is to discuss some important questions for needs assessment researchers to consider in moving from the empirical literature on social support to the design of instruments that utilize this concept. In doing so, the goal is to clarify some alternative ways of conceptualizing and measuring social support. This discussion serves as an introduction to a study that was conducted with a sample of young mothers. The study not only illustrates the use of support measures in assessing the needs of this high risk group, but it also addresses methodological and substantive issues concerning support's stress moderating effects. The implications of this research for the planning of preventive interventions will be discussed.

Conceptual Considerations

One of the basic problems that characterizes much of the literature on social support is the lack of clarity in the social support concept itself (Cohen & McKay, in press; Heller, 1979; Heller &

Swindle, in press). This lack of clarity stems partially from individual reports that fail to define support or provide definitions that are so all-encompassing that the concept loses distinctiveness. Those definitions that have been articulated present some additional confusion because of their diversity and the resultant lack of a consensual conceptualization. An analysis of some of the more prominent descriptions of social support reveals three important distinctions (Barrera & Ainlay, Note 1).

1. Conceptualizations vary on the diversity and breadth of social exchanges that are regarded as falling within the realm of social support. For example, some include the provision of material goods in their descriptions of legitimate support functions while others do not.

2. Some definitions are tied closely to the concept of life stress such that support is viewed as a resource that is primarily accessed for coping with crises. Others have a more noncrisis orientation that includes activities that are involved in socializing and non-problem focused interactions.

3. Support can be defined from the vantage point of the environment such as when it is defined in terms of observable helping behaviors. It can also be defined phenomenologically such as when an individual's perceptions of the availability or adequacy of support is the focus.

There is no correct way of defining social support or no prescriptive solution for selecting among the alternative ways in which it has been conceptualized. Instead, needs assessment planners are faced with the task of first becoming aware of the conceptual alternatives that exist, selecting a conceptualization that is most appropriate to the assessment task, and then communicating this decision in subsequent reports of needs assessment findings.

Even after arriving at a clear definition of social support, there is still an additional conceptual question to be addressed prior to the identification of social support instruments. Like other psychological constructs, social support can be thought to have a variety of properties. Properties such as the number of support providers, frequency of support provision, perceived availability, and others have all been suggested as relevant topics for investigation (cf. Sandler & Barrera, Note 2). The method of social network analysis itself yields a number of properties (Mitchell & Trickett, 1980) that might constitute foci of study for needs assessments.

It seems unlikely that all properties of social support will prove to be equally as relevant for the prevention of certain categories of disorder. However, at the present time there is insufficient research evidence to specify properties of support that consistently moderate life stress or bear direct relationships to physical or psychological symptomatology. As a result, needs assessment researchers must rely on their own judgments in identifying central support properties of their studies.

Measurement Issues

Beyond conceptual decisions that face needs assessment researchers are issues concerning the measurement of social support. A review of early studies on this topic identified the absence of measures with acceptable psychometric properties as a pressing need (Dean & Lin, 1977). For many measures used in this initial research, two limitations were evident. First, the contents of some measures of "social support" were quite heterogeneous. In discussing this point, Heller and Swindle (in press) noted how the heterogeneity of certain measures actually represented a confounding of support with concepts such as personal adjustment and intrapersonal characteristics (e.g., ego strength, self-esteem).

Second, rather global measures of the availability of significant social relationships such as marital status (Eaton, 1978) and the presence of an older sibling (Sandler, 1980) have been used, but these indices fall short of assessing the needs of individuals in a way that will aid the planning of preventive interventions. Gottlieb (1981) commented on the inadequacies of information based on measures of "social embeddedness" by remarking that:

> These data tell us nothing about the number and kind of social contacts associated with low-risk status, or about the interpersonal processes that may lie at the heart of social support. Certainly, these data provide none of the details necessary to inform the design of preventive programs involving the mobilization of social support. (p. 205)

Researchers have, however, recently made substantial improvements in the measurement of social support. Several newly developed scales are measures of individuals' perceived availability of support from various sources, e.g., friends, family members, and colleagues (Holahan & Moos, 1981; Turner, 1981; Cohen & Hoberman, Note 3; Procidano & Heller, Note 4). These instruments have reliabilities well within acceptable limits and have shown meaningful relationships to measures of psychological and psychosocial adjustment.

Measures of other important features of support have also been developed. One scale, the Inventory of Socially Supportive Behaviors (ISSB), was designed to measure the frequency of helping transactions that individuals receive (Barrera, Sandler, & Ramsay, 1981). In one study, the ISSB demonstrated stress-buffering effects for subjects with internal locus of control orientations (Sandler & Lakey, 1982), but in other studies it did not show positive stress buffering effects (Barrera, 1981; Sandler & Barrera, Note 2; Cohen & Hoberman, Note 3).

Two other scales, the Arizona Social Support Interview Schedule (ASSIS) (Barrera, 1980) and the Social Support Questionnaire (Sarason, Levine, Basham, & Sarason, Note 5), require subjects to identify social support network members and also measure their level of satisfaction with support provided. Initial assessment of the scales' psychometric properties showed them to be promising approaches for measuring support.

Because of the recent scale development research, needs assessment investigators are no longer constrained in their selection of scales or properties of support to assess. In fact, there are at least two good reasons for investigators to employ multiple measures of support. As previously mentioned, there is insufficient evidence to a priori select a single property of support as a likely preventive agent of certain forms of disorder for certain populations. In the present developmental stage of this research, exploratory study of several support properties is justifiable and desirable. Second, the simultaneous use of several support measures will increase our understanding of the interrelationships between properties of support. Support measures have not always showed high correlations with each other in the few studies that have used multiple measures. For example, Wilcox (1981) expressed some surprise at finding only a moderate relationship between a measure of the quality of an individual's network and a measure of the quantity of support providers. In two studies (Barrera, 1981; Sandler & Barrera, Note 2) the measure of support satisfaction from the ASSIS was uncorrelated with measures of total network size and the ISSB, while these latter two measures were only mildly correlated with each other.

The use of prospective designs has importance for advancing our understanding of support as a potential prevention agent. Previous studies on the stress-moderating effects of support have typically adopted a "slice-of-time" approach in which stressful events, social support, and adjustment were concurrently assessed (e.g., Barrera, 1981; LaRocco, House, & French, 1980; Sandler, 1980; Wilcox, 1981). With this design the relationship of stress and support to maladjustment cannot be unambiguously interpreted. Conceptual models portray social support and stress as affecting adjustment (e.g., Dohrenwend, 1978), but states of adjustment could conceivably influence perceptions of support and stress as well (cf. Henderson, Byrne, Duncan-Jones, Adcock, Scott, & Steele, 1978). Several authors have advocated the use of longitudinal designs to disentangle the relationships between stress, support, and symptoms (Carveth & Gottlieb, 1979; Dean & Lin, 1977; Dohrenwend & Dohrenwend, 1978; Heller & Swindle, in press).

Background to the Present Study

The present study illustrates the use of multiple measures of social support and a prospective design in which stress and support are assessed prior to the measurement of adjustment. In the tradition of other studies of social support, this research was conducted with a group undergoing a major life transition, i.e., pregnant teenagers. Pregnancy per se is viewed as a major life change as indicated by its presence on several stressful life events scales (Dohrenwend, Krasnoff, Askenasy, & Dohrenwend, 1978; Holmes & Rahe, 1967; Sarason, Johnson, & Siegel, 1978). For teenagers, pregnancy is perceived as particularly stressful (Coddington, 1972) and is associated with a number of physical and social impairments (Card & Wise, 1978; Furstenberg & Crawford, 1978).

There have been some previous investigations of support's stress moderating effects among pregnant women. In a study that is frequently cited as support for the stress-buffering hypothesis, Nuckolls et al. (1972) found that women who reported high life stress and low levels of "psychosocial assets" had three times more birth complications than those women who reported high levels of "psychosocial assets." However, the heterogeneity of their asset measure made it difficult to attribute these effects solely to the influence of social support. Another study by Lewis and Jones (Note 6) reported preliminary results from a sample of 45 unwed pregnant teenagers. For the 24 women who had given birth, prenatal life stress and social support were examined as possible predictors of delivery complications. High support was associated with fewer delivery problems for those women who experienced high stress. For those who reported low stress there were no differences between the high and low support groups. Curiously, women who reported low stress and high support had the same degree of delivery problems as those women with high stress and low support.

The present research follows from a study conducted by the first author (Barrera, 1981). In this initial study, an ethnically diverse sample of adolescents completed life stress, psychological adjustment, and several social support measures during pregnancy. Results showed that one social support index, social network size, demonstrated the predicted stress moderating effects when depression served as the indicator of psychological adjustment. Satisfaction with support was directly related to measures of psychological adjustment.

While this first study dealt with psychological adjustment during pregnancy, the present study is concerned with physical health indicators related to birth outcome. Specifically, the three support variables of network size, satisfaction with support, and frequency of supportive behavioral transactions were examined as predictors of birth complications at delivery. Although the support measures were known to be relatively independent of each other, they were each expected to moderate the relationship between prenatal stressful life events and birth outcome.

METHOD

Subjects

Birth records were located for 74 of the 86 subjects who participated in initial assessments during their pregnancies. The final sample was comprised of 20 blacks, 28 European-Americans, 22 Mexican-Americans, and 4 who identified themselves as members of other ethnic/racial groups. They were a mean of 17.2 years old and had completed an average of 10.9 years of schooling. Twenty-one of the seventy-four subjects were married.

Subjects included in this study were compared with those whose birth records could not be located on a number of demographic, support, stress, and psychological adjustment measures. Only one of these comparisons was significant. Missing subjects ($M = 6.2$) reported significantly more prenatal stressful events that those subjects ($M = 4.1$) in the current study, $t(84) = 2.32, p < .05$.

Procedure

Prenatal assessments were conducted by eight female research assistants[1] who solicited volunteer subjects in two urban agencies that offered special education and health services to pregnant adolescents.[2] Participation was restricted to women who were less than 20 years old and who did not have children from previous pregnancies. At the time of assessment, subjects were a mean of 6.7 months pregnant. The assessment battery consisted of self-report scales and other measures that were administered in structured interviews which typically required one hour. Information concerning birth outcome was obtained from birth records filed with the state's office of vital records. These records were compiled from standard information that hospitals were required to submit for every delivery that was performed.

Measures

Social support. Three social support measures were administered. The psychometric properties of these scales are detailed in several reports (Barrera, 1980, 1981; Barrera et al., 1981). The Inventory of Socially Supportive Behaviors (ISSB) is a 40-item self-report scale for assessing the frequency with which subjects received specific forms of support during the preceding 4-week period (Barrera et al., 1981). In the present study, the ISSB yielded an internal consistency reliability of .92. The Arizona Social Support Interview Schedule (ASSIS) is a structured interview which contains two separate measures (Barrera, 1980). First, it includes procedures for identifying the network of significant others who are providers of social support (total network size). In a previous study (Barrera, 1980), the test-retest reliability of network size was found to be .88. Additionally, subjects make global ratings of their satisfaction with the support that they received during the preceding month (support satisfaction). The support satisfaction scale showed an internal consistency reliability of .50 in the present study.

---

[1]Research assistants in this study were Sally DesCamp, Robyn Kay, Stephanie McFarland, Debbie Martinez, Jean Masciangelo, Carole Maynard, Linda Williams, and Jody Falk who also served as study coordinator.

[2]One agency was an alternative high school for pregnant students who elected to transfer from their home campuses. The second was a public health clinic that provided special pre- and postnatal clinics for teenaged women. Each participant received $3 following the completion of the interview.

Negative life events. A measure of negative life events consisted of 27 undesirable events taken from Coddington's (1972) scale for senior high school students and an additional 8 items concerning victimization from violence and drug use that were written specifically for this study. Interviewers asked subjects to indicate which events had occurred during the preceding six months.

Psychological symptomatology. The Brief Symptom Inventory (BSI) is a self-administered short form of the SCL-90 (Derogatis, 1977). A variety of symptom dimensions such as anxiety, depression, paranoia, interpersonal sensitivity, and somatization are represented in the BSI.

Birth outcome measures. Birth records contained information on prenatal medical care, Apgar scores at 1 and 5 minutes, and indices of pregnancy and birth complications. Two measures were examined in the present study: 1 minute Apgar ratings and the presence (or absence) of birth complications. Other indices proved to be unsuitable because of their low frequency of occurrence.[3]

RESULTS

As shown in Table 1, the only significant relationship between the support measures was the small correlation between total network size and the ISSB. Support satisfaction was not related to these two measures. Distinct relationships between negative life events and support measures were observed. Whereas the measure of negative life events was *positively* correlated with the ISSB, $r(72) = .34$, $p < .01$, it was negatively correlated with support satisfaction, $r(72) = -.38$, $p < .001$, and not correlated with network size, $r(72) = .09$, NS.

Correlations between the birth outcome measures and three subject background characteristics—age, last grade completed, and marital status—were all nonsignificant. Similarly, there were no ethnic group differences on birth outcome measures.

Table 2 shows zero-order correlations between the five predictor variables and birth outcome indices. BSI scores were significantly correlated with Apgar scores, $r(72) = -.26$, $p < .01$, while negative life events was the only significant predictor of birth com-

---

[3]Over 85% of the sample had Apgar scores (at 5 minutes) of 9 or 10, over 90% had no recorded complications of pregnancy, and over 95% had no evidence of significant illnesses during pregnancy.

TABLE 1

Intercorrelations of Prenatal Predictor Variables

Predictor Variables	2	3	4	5
1. Total Network Size	.27**	.00	.09	-.01
2. ISSB		-.12	.34**	.16
3. Support Satisfaction			-.38***	-.50***
4. Negative Life Events				.33**
5. BSI -- Total Symptoms				

$\underline{N}$ = 74

   *$\underline{p}$ < .05

 **$\underline{p}$ < .01

***$\underline{p}$ < .001

plications, $r(72) = .24$, $p < .05$. None of the social support measures were directly related to either outcome variable.

As a test of the stress-buffering hypothesis, each of the criterion measures were regressed on stressful life events, social support and interaction terms created by multiplying stress and support scores. Of the six hierarchical regression analyses that were subsequently conducted, one was significant. In the regression analyses of Apgar scores neither the independent effects of negative events nor network size was statistically significant. However, the interaction term, $F(1,70) = 4.07, p < .05$, as well as the combined effects of the predictors, $F(3.70) = 2.87, p < .05$, were significant.

As an aid in interpreting this interaction, the overall sample was divided at the median to form high and low support groups. Within each of these subsamples, negative life events and Apgar scores were correlated.[4] As shown in Table 3 the predicted relationships were obtained; negative life events were significantly correlated

---

[4]Since the variance of scores within each subsample can effect the magnitude of correlations, tests for homogeneity of variance were conducted for all stress and birth outcome measures for all pairs of subsamples. One significant difference was noted. For Apgar scores at 1 minute, there was less variability in the high support satisfaction group than there was for the low support satisfaction group.

with Apgar scores for women with small support networks, $r(33) = -.37$, but not for those with large networks, $r(37) = .09$, NS. Parallel analyses were also conducted for the ISSB and the support satisfaction measure. Table 3 shows that the results for support satisfaction and birth complications were also consistent with the stress-buffering hypothesis. For women who reported low satisfaction with the support they received during their pregnancies, negative life events were moderately correlated with birth complications, $r(34) = .42, p < .01$; these variables were not significantly

TABLE 2

Correlations Between Prenatal Predictor Variables

and Birth Outcome Indicators

Predictor Variable	Apgar [a] (1 min.)	Birth Complications
Total Network Size	.17	.00
ISSB	-.08	.18
Support Satisfaction	.19	-.09
Negative Life Events	-.15	.24*
BSI -- Total Symptoms	-.26**	.15

Note: $\underline{N}$ = 74

[a]Apgar scores are based on ratings of medical personnel who observe the infant at one and five minutes following delivery. Ratings of 0, 1, or 2 are assigned to each of five categories: heart rate, respiratory effort, muscle tone, reflex irritability, and skin color.

Total scores represent the sum of the five category ratings with higher scores indicating greater heartiness. Scores of 7-10 are typically regarded as "normal".

 *$\underline{p}$ < .05

**$\underline{p}$ < .01

TABLE 3

Correlations Between Negative Life Events and

Birth Outcome Indicators for High and Low Support Groups

			r	N	Z
Apgar (1 min.)					
1. Total Network Size		Low	-.37*	35	1.97*
		High	.09	39	
2. ISSB		Low	-.02	36	NS
		High	-.24	38	
3. Support Satisfaction[a]		Low	-.19	36	NS
		High	.07	38	
Birth Complications					
1. Total Network Size		Low	.19	35	NS
		High	.29	39	
2. ISSB		Low	.16	36	NS
		High	.26	38	
3. Support Satisfaction		Low	.42**	36	1.64*
		High	.05	38	

[a]There was significantly less variability in Apgar scores for the high support group than for the low support group.

*p < .05

**p < .01

correlated for women who reported high satisfaction, $r(36) = .05$, NS.

DISCUSSION

This prospective study offers support for the proposition that properties of social support moderate the relationship of negative life events to birth outcomes of teenage mothers. The design and methods used in this study overcame some ambiguities of the initial investigation with these subjects (Barrera, 1981) and other non-prospective studies of the stress-buffering hypothesis. Unlike a number of studies on this topic, (a) not all measures were self-report instruments since the major criterion variables were based on medical records, (b) outcome criteria were measured several months following the assessment of both life events and social support, and (c) multiple measures of support were included in the assessment battery. As Heller and Swindle (in press) asserted, cross-sectional correlational studies of social support's stress buffering effects can make only a limited contribution to what we already know. If social support is to be promoted as a viable concept for the development of preventive interventions, additional prospective research is needed, particularly research that does not rely entirely on self-report for the measurement of outcome criteria.

While it would be unjustifiable to generalize these results to other groups undergoing different life transitions, this study does illustrate how measures of support can be incorporated into needs assessment research and how resultant findings can guide the design of interventions. In the present study, both total support network size and support satisfaction emerged as significant predictors. However, network size entered into the prediction of the relatively transient criterion variable of Apgar ratings. Support satisfaction, on the other hand, was related to complications at delivery and also showed the strongest relationships to scales of psychological adjustment in the initial study of this sample. While both support variables constitute reasonable targets for intervention, the present investigation points to support satisfaction as the most relevant yardstick for measuring the adequacy of a preventive intervention for this subpopulation.

The inclusion of several distinct support measures made it possible to examine the relationship between them. Similar to the results of a previous study with college students (Sandler & Barrera, Note 2), network size and frequency of supportive behaviors were uncorrelated with support satisfaction ratings. Although support satisfaction emerged as the most salient predictor of birth complications and psychological symptomatology, neither the overall number of support providers nor the amount of supportive behavioral exchanges appeared to be related to satisfaction ratings. These findings suggest that innovative intervention methods will have to move beyond the manipulation of network size and frequency of support in order to impact on individuals' subjective evaluations of satisfaction with the support that they receive.

To maintain the appropriate context for this illustrative study, two points deserve emphasis. First, social support is only one of several factors that might have been studied in the present research, and certainly, support is only one of several factors that have importance for understanding the physical and psychological well-being of young mothers. Placing social support within a broader "multiple factorial causality" model of the targets of preventive interventions will aid in restraining the portrayal of support as a panacea (Heller, Price, & Sher, 1980). Second, there are dangers in concluding that the support variables that did or did not predict the outcome criteria used in the present study will do the same in subsequent studies of different samples, life transitions, and outcome criteria.

Despite some continuing differences in the way social support is conceptualized, there have been gains in the measurement of various support properties, most notably in the assessment of the perceived availability of support. As a result, needs assessment researchers have a number of alternatives for measuring diverse aspects of support. This study and others have pointed out how measures of distinct aspects of support are not always highly correlated. One implication of this observation is that very different conclusions about the needs of populations and subsequent preventive interventions can be reached depending on the assessment approaches that are adopted. While social support appears to deserve a place in both needs assessments and preventive interventions, there is still a relatively thin data base that can be cited as evidence of support's preventive effects. Building preventive interventions around social support concepts will obviously not be appropriate under all circumstances. The critical contribution of needs assessments is in providing an empirical basis for identifying when certain properties of support are relevant for certain subpopulations. The challenges that face social support researchers include the development of instruments that inform the design of prevention programs and the implementation of more action research that will demonstrate the efficacy of preventive interventions that are built on social support principles.

REFERENCE NOTES

1. Barrera, M., Jr., & Ainlay, S.L. *The structure of social support: A conceptual and empirical analysis.* Unpublished manuscript, Arizona State University, 1981.

2. Sandler, I.N., & Barrera, M., Jr. *Social support as a stress-buffer: A multi-method investigation.* Paper presented at the meeting of the American Psychological Association, Montreal, August 1980.

3. Cohen, S., & Hoberman, H. *Life events, social support and self-reported symptoms: Buffering life change.* Unpublished manuscript, University of Oregon, 1981.

4. Procidano, M.E., & Heller, K. *Toward the assessment of perceived social support.* Paper presented at the meeting of the American Psychological Association, New York, 1979.

5. Sarason, I.G., Levine, H.M., Basham, R.B., & Sarason, B.R. *Assessing social support: The Social Support Questionnaire* (Tech. Rep. CO-004). Seattle: University of Washington, Department of Psychology, May 1981.
6. Lewis, J.D., & Jones, A.C. *Psychological stress, social support systems, and pregnancy complications in adolescents.* Paper presented at the meeting of the American Psychological Association, Montreal, August 1980.

REFERENCES

Barrera, M., Jr. A method for the assessment of social support networks in community survey research. *Connections,* 1980, *3,* 8-13.

Barrera, M., Jr. Social support in the adjustment of pregnant adolescents: Assessment issues. In B.H. Gottlieb (Ed.), *Social networks and social support in community mental health.* Beverly Hills: Sage, 1981.

Barrera, M., Jr., Sandler, I.N., & Ramsay, T.B. Preliminary development of a scale of social support: Studies on college students. *American Journal of Community Psychology,* 1981, *9,* 435-447.

Bowlby, G. *Attachment.* New York: Basic Books, 1969.

Card, J.J., & Wise, L.L. Teenage mothers and teenage fathers: The impact of early childbearing on the parents' personal and professional lives. *Family Planning Perspectives,* 1978, *10,* 199-235.

Carveth, W.B., & Gottlieb, B.H. The measurement of social support and its relation to stress. *Canadian Journal of Behavioral Science,* 1979, *11,* 179-187.

Coddington, R.D. The significance of life events as etiologic factors in the diseases of children: I-A survey of professional workers. *Journal of Psychosomatic Research,* 1972, *16,* 7-18.

Cohen, S., & McKay, G. Social support, stress and the buffering hypothesis: An empirical review. In A. Baum, J.E. Singer, & S.E. Taylor (Eds.), *Handbook of psychology and health* (Vol. 4). Hillsdale, N.J.: Erlbaum, in press.

Dean, A., & Lin, N. The stress-buffering role of social support. *Journal of Nervous and Mental Disease,* 1977, *165,* 403-417.

Derogatis, L.R. *SCL-90: Administration, scoring, and procedures manual—I for the R version.* Baltimore: Author, 1977.

Dohrenwend, B.S. Social stress and community psychology. *American Journal of Community Psychology,* 1978, *6,* 1-14.

Dohrenwend, B.S., & Dohrenwend, B.P. Some issues in research in stressful life events. *The Journal of Nervous and Mental Disease,* 1978, *166,* 7-15.

Dohrenwend, B.S., Krasnoff, L., Askenasy, A.R., & Dohrenwend, B.P. Exemplification of a method for scaling life events: The PERI life events scale. *Journal of Health and Social Behavior,* 1978, *19,* 205-229.

Eaton, W.W. Life events, social supports, and psychiatric symptoms: A re-analysis of the New Haven data. *Journal of Health and Social Behavior,* 1978, *19,* 230-234.

Furstenberg, F.F., & Crawford, A.G. Family support: Helping teenage mothers to cope. *Family Planning Perspectives,* 1978, *10,* 322-33.

Gottlieb, B.H. Preventive interventions involving social networks and social support. In B.H. Gottlieb (Ed.), *Social networks and social support.* Beverly Hills: Sage, 1981.

Gottlieb, B.H., & Hall, A. Social networks and the utilization of preventive mental health services. In R.H. Price, R.F. Ketterer, B.C. Bader, & J. Monahan (Eds.), *Prevention in mental health: Research, policy, and practice.* Beverly Hills: Sage, 1980.

Gourash, N. Help-seeking: A review of the literature. *American Journal of Community Psychology,* 1978, *6,* 413-23.

Heller, K. The effects of social support: Prevention and treatment implications. In A.P. Goldstein & F.H. Kanfer (Eds.), *Maximizing treatment gains: Transfer enhancement in psychotherapy.* New York: Academic Press, 1979.

Heller, K., Price, R.H., & Sher, K.J. Research and evaluation in primary prevention: Issues and guidelines. In R.H. Price, R.F. Ketterer, B.C. Bader, & J. Monahan (Eds.), *Prevention in mental health: Research, policy, and practice.* Beverly Hills: Sage, 1980.

Heller, K., & Swindle, R.W. Social networks, perceived social support and coping with stress. In R.D. Felner, L.A. Jason, J. Mortisugu, & S.S. Farber (Eds.), *Preventive psychology: Theory, research and practice in community intervention.* New York: Pergamon Press, in press.

Henderson, S. The social network, support and neurosis. *British Journal of Psychiatry,* 1977, *131,* 185-91.

Henderson, S., Byrne, D.G., Duncan-Jones, P., Adcock, S., Scott, R., & Steele, G.P. Social bonds in the epidemiology of neurosis: A preliminary communication. *British Journal of Psychiatry,* 1978, *132,* 463-66.

Holahan, C.J., & Moos, R.H. Social support and psychological distress: A longitudinal analysis. *Journal of Abnormal Psychology,* 1981, *90,* 365-70.

Holmes, T.H., & Rahe, R.H. The social readjustment rating scale. *Psychosomatic Medicine,* 1967, *11,* 213-218.

LaRocco, J.M., House, J.S., & French, J.R.P. Social support occupational stress and health. *Journal of Health and Social Behavior,* 1980, *21,* 202-218.

Nuckolls, K.B., Cassel, J., & Kaplan, B.H. Psychosocial assets, life crises and the prognosis of pregnancy. *American Journal of Epidemiology,* 1972, *95,* 431-441.

Sandler, I.N. Social support resources, stress and maladjustment of poor children. *American Journal of Community Psychology,* 1980, *8,* 41-52.

Sandler, I.N., & Lakey, B. Locus of control as a stress moderator: The role of control perceptions and social support. *American Journal of Community Psychology,* 1982, *10,* 65-80.

Sarason, I.G., Johnson, J.H., & Siegel, J.M. Assessing the impact of life changes: Development of the life experiences survey. *Journal of Consulting and Clinical Psychology,* 1978, *46,* 932-46.

Turner, R.J. Social support as a contingency in psychological well-being. *Journal of Health and Social Behavior,* 1981, *22,* 357-67.

Weiss, R.S. The fund of sociability. *TransAction,* 1969, *6,* 36-43.

Wilcox, B.L. Social support, life stress, and psychological adjustment: A test of the buffering hypothesis. *American Journal of Community Psychology,* 1981, *9,* 371-86.

Needs Assessment
and Community Development:
An Ideological Perspective

Sylvia Martí-Costa
Irma Serrano-García

ABSTRACT. Many practitioners of the social sciences have fostered the value-free, apolitical and ahistorical character of their disciplines. This position distorts the real perception that should permeate the theory, methodology, techniques and practices of the social sciences. This paper, by examining the method of needs assessment, focuses on the undesirability of preserving this point of view. Needs assessment is discussed as a political process for the organization, mobilization and consciousness-raising of groups and communities.

Community development is a process which, through consciousness-raising, promotes and utilizes human resources, leading to the empowerment of individuals and communities so that they can understand and solve their problems and create new circumstances for their livelihood. As part of this process, needs assessment may be utilized as a central method to facilitate the modification of social systems so they become more responsive to human needs.

At the individual level, community development promotes psychological growth and enhancement by channeling energies into self-help projects and through the genuine participation of individuals in those decisions that affect their lives. The basic assumption that underlies this reasoning is that most human beings can solve their problems when they obtain access to resources and create alternatives. The emphasis is on their strengths and their development (Rappaport, 1977).

Awareness of problems and of change possibilities is achieved by

---

Reprints may be obtained from Irma Serrano-García, Department of Psychology, University of Puerto Rico, Río Piedras, Puerto Rico 00931.

75

raising an individual's consciousness from its current or real level to its possible capacity. Real consciousness is defined as an individual or groups' understanding of reality at a given time. Possible consciousness is the maximum understanding that can be achieved by an individual or group according to its material circumstances at a given historical moment (Goldman, 1970).

Consciousness-raising includes critical judgment of situations, the search for underlying causes of problems and their consequences, and an active role in the transformation of society (Ander-Egg, 1980). It is an awareness of human dignity and is essential in the exploration of the relationship between the social order and human misery and in the discovery of the shortcomings inherent in our society (Freire, 1974). It facilitates individual and collective participation in building a new and less oppressive social order, thus affecting the general well-being of the population by enhancing the relationship between individuals and society. Needs assessment is valuable in the consciousness-raising process, because any social movement should start from and respond to the felt needs of the population, in other words, their real consciousness.

Community development can foster consciousness-raising through the involvement of individuals in change efforts. Community development activities need to be grounded in a specific political commitment that responds to the liberation of the powerless groups of society. This does not ignore the participation of the powerful in the maintenance or change of the present social order. It does, however, require a personal and professional commitment to the oppressed because of the mission of prevention—understanding and relieving human suffering.

Contrary to this view, many social scientists have fostered the value-free, apolitical, and ahistorical character of their disciplines throughout several decades (Moscovici, 1972; Weimer, 1979; Zuñiga, 1975). This position, which may be referred to as "the myth of neutrality," distorts the real value-laden and political nature of theory, methods, and practices and thus serves to alienate us from ourselves and others (Ander-Egg, 1973). It creates divisions and distrust within our ranks and resentment from those that participate as "subjects" or recipients of our work, feeling used, manipulated and misunderstood. Thus, it is necessary to examine this myth which has resulted in the social sciences serving the dominant groups of society.

The "myth of neutrality" has reasons for its existence. In some cases it has been sponsored by individuals who clearly believe in it, but in most cases, it has been accepted inadvertently by social scientists. One of the ways in which this occurs is by considering objectivity and neutrality as synonymous and inseparable concepts which are highly desirable in social scientific endeavors.

Those that hold that neutrality and objectivity must go together state that social scientists should not take political stances toward the object of their studies because this will hamper their research efforts (Myrdal, 1969). To them objectivity is defined as the capacity to study facts as they occur, without adhering to previously formed opinions and judgments and with the willingness to abandon positions that are proven false, inadequate, and unsatisfactory (Ander-Egg, 1977). Neutrality, its inseparable counterpart, is defined as a valueless stance before the objective reality (Martí, Note 1).

It is said that if researchers are not neutral, they cannot be objective (Martí, Note 1). This does not ring true as both concepts are different and clearly distinguishable, and while the pursuit of objectivity is desirable and necessary, the search for neutrality is not only impossible, but unwarranted. Objectivity is desirable because its definition implies the existence of defined values and positions which one is willing to change when an examination of reality requires it. Neutrality is impossible because every activity takes place in a particular political context.

If the political nature of the social sciences is recognized and accepted then an explicit definition of social scientists' values is necessary. It is our position that this value stance must be characterized by a commitment to the disadvantaged and powerless groups within a given society. This commitment is to the abandonment of a spectator role and the activation of a professional's mind and art to the service of a cause (Palau, Note 2). This cause should be the significant transformation of inequities in society which implies activism, risk, initiative, and a willingness to fight for clearly defined points of view.

To summarize, needs assessment is an integral part of community development, the process of consciousness-raising. It implies a political commitment which undermines the traditional view of a neutral science and a firm commitment to the exploited, underprivileged and powerless groups in society.

This paper will show that needs assessment is a political process that can be conceptualized as a tool for the organization, mobilization and consciousness-raising of groups and communities. This implies (1) that the diverse uses of needs assessment methods be placed on a continuum, ranging from the perpetuation of control and the maintenance of the social system to the achievement of radical social change; (2) an emphasis on multiple techniques of needs assessment that facilitate collective activities, leadership development, growth of organizational skills, and participation of community members in interventions within research (Irizarry & Serrano, 1979); and (3) the belief that it is necessary to examine ideologies and values as they influence objectives, the selection of needs assessment techniques, intervention strategies, conceptual frameworks, and the utilization of obtained data.

NEEDS ASSESSMENT

Purpose

Needs assessment is part of a process used to plan social service programs (Pharis, 1976; Siegel, Attkinson, & Cohn, 1977). It is used to determine the problems and goals of the residents of a given community to assure that an intervention will respond to the needs of the population that is being sampled (Warheit, 1976).

The purposes that sustain the use of needs assessment methodology can be placed on a continuum (Table 1) according to their political roles. Towards the top of Table 1 are purposes that foster system maintenance and control; towards the bottom are ones that promote social change and consciousness-raising. Social system maintenance and control efforts include those activities which are carried out to maintain and/or strengthen the status quo. They also include first order change efforts which alter some of the ways in which the system functions but not the ideology on which it is based (Watzlawick, Weakland, & Fisch, 1974). Radical, or second order, social change efforts imply consciousness-raising and structural and functional alterations.

In consonance with these definitions, the very bottom of the continuum shows needs assessment as a mechanism used by community residents for participation and control in decision making. Needs assessment becomes a technique that facilitates second order social change.

The very top of the continuum lists purposes that foster system maintenance and control, including those that are used to obtain ad-

Table 1

Continuum of Needs Assessment Purposes

Political Role	Purpose
Control System Maintenance	- Guarantee the economic survival of service programs
	- Respond to interest group pressures
	- Provide services required by communities
	- Program evaluation
	- Program planning
	- Public policy decision-making
Social Change	- Measure, describe, and understand community life styles
	- Assess community resources to lessen external dependency
	- Return needs assessment data to facilitate residents' decision-making
	- Provide skill training, leadership, and organizational skills
	- Facilitate collective activities and group mobilization
	- Facilitate consciousness-raising

ditional funding for already established community programs (Siegel et al., 1977) so as to guarantee their continuation. In the middle of the continuum, but still focusing on maintenance and control efforts, are included purposes such as (a) planning for decision-making and program evaluation (Murell, 1976); (b) gaining additional input toward personnel recruitment; (c) describing, measuring and understanding different aspects of community life (Siegel et al., 1977); (d) determining discrepancies between residents' and professionals' points of view (Ronald, Titus, Strasser, & Vess, Note 3); and (e) obtaining knowledge about community resources so as to link these to agency services.

In analyzing this continuum it is important to notice that most needs assessment efforts are directed towards consumer satisfaction and agency survival. These are legitimate and necessary goals; however, if technique development is limited to these goals, it will be incomplete and unsatisfactory. Needs assessment methodology, if it is to respond to a commitment to the powerless and to the fostering of social change, must (a) emphasize techniques that, singly or in combination, facilitate grouping and mobilizing people; (b) foster collective activities; (c) facilitate leadership development; and (d) involve residents in the entire research process. These characteristics are essential so that the technique can facilitate consciousness-raising.

Categorization and Evaluation of Techniques

At present there is a great diversity of needs assessment techniques. In some instances it is suggested that different techniques be combined focusing on diverse kinds of interventions (Aponte, 1976; Pharis, 1976; Siegel et al., 1977). Others suggest that only one technique be used with one line of intervention preferred (Clifford, Note 4; Evans, Note 5; Zautra, Note 6). In order to respond to the goals of organization, mobilization, and consciousness-raising in communities, the multiple techique approach is more desirable since a more precise view of reality is obtained. More data is gathered which will vary quantitatively and qualitatively, thus providing a thorough appraisal of community needs. Another reason for the combined use of techniques is that their limitations and deficiencies can be balanced. However, it is also important to study how each individual technique contributes to the goal of greater mobilization.

Needs assessment techniques can be grouped in three different categories defined by the contact they provide between the researcher and community residents. This contact is extremely important as it may be used to foster collectivization, mobilization, leadership development, and resident involvement (Ander-Egg, 1980; Sanguinetti, 1981), characteristics that are essential to a new focus on needs assessment goals.

No contact with participants. In this category, techniques permit no relationship between the intervener and the participants. These techniques are rates or percentages under treatment, social indicators, social area analysis and dynamic modeling (Kleemeir, Stephenson, & Isaacs, Note 7; Bell, 1976; Murell, 1976; Pharis, 1976). In general terms, these methods try to determine community needs by utilizing qualitative and quantitative data from several sources, such as demographic records and other social indicators. They are based on the assumption that community needs and problems that appear in official statistics are representative of community problems. The major limitation of the "non-contact with the participant" techniques lies in their absolute lack of direct mobilization potential. Since the residents are not involved in the needs assessment project—in fact, it can even happen without their knowledge—their involvement in social action efforts is not to be expected.

Contact with the agency or community. The "contact with the agency or community" category includes observation (Ander-Egg, 1978), service provider assessment (Kelly, Note 8), key informants (Pharis, 1976), behavioral census (Murell, 1976), surveys (Clifford, Note 4; O'Brien, Note 9), nominal groups (Delbecq, Van de Ven, & Gustatson, 1975), and community forums (Kleemeir et al., Note 7) among other techniques. The interaction that these techniques allows for takes place basically through three means: observations, interviews, and group meetings.

Observation facilitates interaction by the observer's mere presence in the setting. Interviewers interact individually and in groups with community residents, service providers, or other key informants to directly obtain data. This interaction takes place openly, as in community forums, or in a more controlled manner, as in nominal groups.

Key informants, nominal groups, community forums, and surveys respond to the goals of mobilization and consciousness-raising in the community. The first three techniques encourage community input by eliciting residents' discussions and introspections about the collective nature of their problems and needs. They serve to strengthen communication networks in the community and they facilitate the process of program planning. Survey techniques share some of these qualities if the survey is constructed, coordinated, and administered by community members. This process generates great involvement and knowledge and the ready acceptance of results by the rest of the community (Sanguinetti, 1981).

The nominal group technique has these, and other, advantages. Because of the structured nature of its process (Delbecq et al., 1975), it (1) maximizes the amount, diversity, and quality of the problems and alternatives proposed; (2) inhibits the control of the group by a few vocal persons (Siegel et al., 1977); (3) allows conflicting opinions to be tolerated; (4) fosters creativity; (5) facilitates attention to the contributions of marginal group members; and (6) emphasizes the role of needs assessment as the basis for program creation and planning. These four techniques have the highest mobilization potential.

Combined techniques. This category includes convergent analysis (Bell, 1976), community impressions (Siegel et al., 1977), community meetings/surveys (Kleemeir et al., Note 7), and others. Convergent analysis techniques include techniques of service utilization, social indicators, and surveys. Each technique is used with a specific objective in mind and it is expected that, overall, the information offered by the techniques should give an estimate of those persons whose needs are not being satisfied.

Community impressions and community meetings/surveys have several common elements. The former include the techniques of key informants, data revision, and community forum. The latter includes the first two steps in addition to a survey, allowing the data to be validated and permitting additional verbal input from participants. Although all these techniques require a lot of energy and effort, they are the best alternative in the needs assessment process because they combine high mobilization potential with the more traditional criteria of representativity, validity, and reliability.

Criteria to Judge the Adequacy of Techniques

Given the diversity of techniques, it is necessary to develop specific factors or criteria that should be considered in judging the adequacy of a technique. Some authors have examined this issue and have proposed criteria for the selection of techniques. These criteria include: the nature of the problem, the skills of both the researcher and the participants, available resources (League of California Cities, 1979), representativeness, the specificity required of the information (Murell, 1976), and the amount of political risk that the sponsoring group desires to tolerate (Aponte, 1976).

Although all these criteria are useful, additional criteria should be considered if the needs assessment effort is to contribute to community organization and mobilization. These criteria are presented in Table 2 and contrasted with more traditional views. The following dimensions are used as a guideline for this comparison: the goals, sources, content, and processes of the assessment.

A major distinction between the two sets of criteria is their goals. One set emphasizes prevention and promotion and the awareness of the collective nature of needs. The other works from a remedial

Table 2

Suggested Criteria to Evaluate the Adequacy
of Needs Assessment Techniques

| | Criteria | |
Dimensions of Needs Assessment Process	Criteria that foster mobilization	Traditional Criteria
Goals of Assessment	Prevention and Promotion	Treatment
	Awareness of collective nature of needs	Individual focus
	Encourage collective action	Foster dependency on external resources
Source of Input	Community residents Marginal groups	Service providers Total population
Content of Assessment	All perceived needs Internal community resources	Assessment of needed services
Processes of Assessment	Facilitate community involvement and control of process	Assessment carried out by "experts"
	Facilitate face to face interaction between intervener researcher and participants	Lack of community participation Interaction highly controlled by scientific standards
	Data belongs to participants	Data collection and future planning controlled by agencies
	Planning and collective action carried out by intervener-researcher and participants	

perspective which focuses on the individual and on fostering dependency on external resources. The impact of these differences is most noticeable in the assessment process since a collective focus requires a collective intervention and an individual focus does not.

An evaluation of previously mentioned techniques according to the community organization and mobilization criteria appears in Table 3. As can be seen, key informants, surveys, nominal groups and community forums are the most adequate techniques. It is important to stress, however, that no single technique can be seen as valid for all times and circumstances; therefore, they should be

Table 3

Evaluation of Needs Assessment Techniques According to their
Potential for Mobilization, Organization and Consciousness-Raising

T e c h n i q u e s

Criteria	Social Records	Computer Use	Observation	Social Indicators	Dynamic Modelling	Systems Model	Surveys	Key Informants	Forum	Nominal Group	Service Provider Assessments	Behavioral Census	Key Persons
Obtains information from community residents							X		X	X			X
Obtains information from marginal groups	X						X		X	X			X
Achieves change in services provided			X				X	X	X	X	X	X	X
Facilitates identifying a wide range of needs		X	X	X			X		X	X			
Facilitates development of internal resources								X	X	X		X	X
Control of information by residents			X	X			X	X	X	X		X	X
Oriented toward prevention			X					X	X				
Collective view of problems								X	X				
Committment to residents' participation in general								X	X				
Committment to residents' participation in research							X	X	X				
a. data collection							X	X	X				
b. instrument construction							X	X	X				X
c. data analysis							X	X	X				X
d. data returns								X	X				X
Fosters Relationship between residents and intervener								X	X	X			X
a. more time together							X	X	X				X
b. dialogue							X	X	X				X
Facilitate collective activities								X	X				X
a. two or more persons								X	X				
b. two or more persons regarding common problems								X	X				
c. adding the discussion of possible solutions								X	X				
d. initiate collective action								X	X				

tailored to the particular situation in which the needs assessment is conducted.

NEEDS ASSESSMENT AND COMMUNITY DEVELOPMENT

Irizarry and Serrano (1979) have developed a model, Intervention within Research, which integrates needs assessment into a community development approach. It uses needs assessment as its methodological foundation and the concept of problematization as its ideological guideline (Freire, 1974). Problematization, our translation for the term *problematización,* refers to the process whereby consciousness-raising takes place. If the latter is seen as the goal, then problematization involves the different strategies whereby it can be achieved.

The model conceptualizes the processes of intervention and research as simultaneous and interdependent. It also assumes that all phases of the model should be permeated with explicit ideological inputs that lead to consciousness-raising.

The objectives suggested for this model include: (1) the creation of collective efforts to solve community problems as defined by community residents; (2) the achievement of individual and group participation in the analysis of social reality; (3) the creation of grass-roots organizations; and (4) the development of political skills among participants, resulting in their increased involvement in public affairs.

The model includes four phases. The first phase, familiarization with the community, includes a review of all written and statistical material regarding the community, and several visits to the same. This approach provides knowledge regarding the community's history, its structures, and the processes which facilitate the intervener's entry into the community. It should emphasize the early identification of key persons in the community through informal communication or through more structured means.

The second phase, which arises from a later revision of the original model (Martí, Note 1), is characterized by the creation of a core group that must be composed of both key community persons and interveners. This core group has planning, coordination, and evaluation responsibilities throughout the entire process of intervention within research.

The creation of this core group has positive psychological and operative repercussions. Since the group is formed with community people, a more effective dialogue can take place. It is also possible to increase their commitment and guarantee the group's continuance in this way. In addition, the key person can acquire skills through modeling or training that will be useful to future community work.

One of the most important tasks of this group is the direction and coordination of the needs assessment. This begins with the core group taking an active role in evaluating the relevance of the different needs assessment techniques to their particular community.

The group's next step is the consideration of alternative actions to develop an effective propaganda campaign to inform residents of the needs assessment. In this effort it is essential to obtain the support of other organized groups in the community.

The core group should direct the needs assessment process per se as well as the process of returning the analyzed data to community residents. This can be done through letters, individual visits, group meetings, or community assemblies. The method used will be determined by the needs assessment technique previously used, by the number of participants it entailed, and by the number of human resources available. The data should be returned promptly and should be explained in simple terms.

The third phase, formation of task groups, includes group activities suggested by the needs assessment. In this phase, short and long term goals are defined and further action plans developed. To carry out these activities an organizational structure must be created. It is suggested that for this purpose a general community meeting should be held where task groups are formed around the needs assessment priorities. This general meeting should be planned and conducted by all participants with the support and guidance of the core group.

In addition to the task groups, workshops and other social, cultural, educational, and recreational activities must be fostered. Workshops should concentrate on the development of skills so as to help community groups deal effectively with outside forces that rally against their efforts. Some possible topics for the workshops are leadership, skills to deal with service agencies, interpersonal communication, propaganda, and organizational skills. Particular attention should be given to internal group processes so that the task groups decision-making will improve, their leadership struggles diminish, and their cohesiveness increase. We believe that this last characteristic is particularly important and that both the workshops and group tasks should emphasize cohesiveness.

The last phase in the model, involvement of new groups, is initiated after some of the short and long term goals of the task groups are achieved. This involves the development of new goals which should help in bringing together other community groups. The steps described should be repeated in a cyclical manner because needs change throughout the process and the community may develop other goals and interests.

CONCLUSION

This paper has presented an alternative ideological framework to evaluate and direct needs assessment efforts. It has also presented a model for its use for community development. Community residents can and should control intervention within research efforts that directly or indirectly involve them and scientists should facilitate this control. If some of these changes are incorporated into current needs assessment efforts, scientists will be more responsive to the people to whom their major efforts should be directed.

REFERENCE NOTES

1. Martí, S. *Hacia una identificación de necesidades en el sector femenino del Barrio Buen Consejo*. Unpublished M.A. thesis, University of Puerto Rico, 1980.
2. Palau, A. *La investigación con la técnica de observación: ¿Para quién y desde dónde?* Unpublished manuscript, 1977. (Avaliable at Sociology Department, University of Puerto Rico, Río Piedras, P.R.).
3. Ronald, L., Titus, W., Stasser, G., & Vess, J. *Views of mental health: A first step in needs assessment*. Paper presented at the 87th Annual Convention of the American Psychological Association. New York City, 1979.
4. Clifford, D.L. *A critical view of need assessment in community mental health planning*. Paper presented at the Second National Conference on Needs Assessment in Health and Human Services, Louisville, Kentucky, 1978.
5. Evans, P. *A model for conducting needs assessment and a report on national ratios*. Paper presented at the 87th Annual Convention of the American Psychological Association, New York City, 1979.
6. Zautra, A. *Quality of life determinants: Some guidelines for measuring community well-being*. Paper presented at the Second National Conference on Need Assessment in Health and Human Services, Louisville, Kentucky, March, 1978.
7. Kleemeir, C.P., Stephenson, D.P., & Isaacs, L.D. *Developing a needs assessment approach for community consultation and education*. Paper presented at the 87th Annual Convention of the American Psychological Association, New York City, 1979.
8. Kelly, M. *Halton region services for children: A needs assessment*. Unpublished manuscript, 1978. (Available at Faculty of Social Work, Wilfrid Laurier University, Waterloo, Ontario, Canada).
9. O'Brien, D. *Merging the technical and community catalytic functions of citizen surveys: Toward a theoretical framework*. Paper presented at the Second National Conference on Needs Assessment in Health and Human Services, Louisville, Kentucky, 1978.

REFERENCES

Ander-Egg, E. *Hacia una metodología de la militancia y el compromiso*. Buenos Aires: Ecro, 1973.
Ander-Egg, E. *Diccionario del trabajo social*. Barcelona: Nova Terra, 1977.
Ander-Egg, E. *Introducción a las técnicas de investigación social*. Buenos Aires: Humanitas, 1978.

Ander-Egg, E. *Metodología del desarrollo de comunidad.* Madrid: UNIEUROP, 1980.
Aponte, S.F. Implications for the future of need assessment. In R.A. Bell, M. Sundel, S.F. Aponte, & S.A. Murell (Eds.), *Needs assessment in health and human services.* Louisville: University of Louisville, 1976.
Bell, R.A. The use of a convergent assessment model in the determination of health status and assessment of need. In R.S. Bell, M. Sundel, J.F. Aponte, & S.A. Murell (Eds.), *Needs assessment in health and human services.* Louisville: University of Louisville, 1976.
Delbecq, A., Van de Ven, H., & Gustatson, D. *Group techniques for program planning: A guide to nominal group and delphi processes.* Chicago: Scott, Foresman, & Company, 1975.
Freire, P. *Pedagogía del oprimido.* México: Siglo 21, 1974.
Goldman, L. Conciencia adecuada, conciencia posible y conciencia falsa. In L. Goldman (Ed.), *Marxismo y ciencias humanas.* Paris: Galiemard, 1970.
Irizarry, A., & Serrano-García, I. Intervención en la investigación: Su aplicación al Barrio Buen Consejo. *Boletín AVEPSO,* 1979, *2,* 6-21.
League of California Cities. Social needs assessment: A scientific or political process. In F. Cox, J. Erlich, J. Rothman, & J. Trafman (Eds.), *Strategies of community organization.* Tasca, Illinois: F.E. Peacock, 1979.
Moscovici, S. Society and theory in social psychology. In J. Israel & H. Tajfel (Eds.), *The context of social psychology.* New York: Academic Press, 1972.
Murell, S.A. Eight process steps for converting needs assessment data into program operations. In S.A. Bell, M. Sundel, J. Aponte, & S. Murell (Eds.), *Needs assessment in health and human services.* Louisville: University of Louisville, 1976.
Myrdal, G. *Objectivity in social research.* New York: Random House, 1969.
Pharis, D.B. The use of needs assessment techniques in mental health planning. *Community Mental Health Review,* 1976, *1,* 4-11.
Rappaport, J. *Community psychology: Values, research and action.* New York: Holt, Rinehart, & Winston, 1977.
Sanguinetti, Y. La investigación participativa en los procesos de desarrollo de américa latina. *Revista de ALAPSO,* 1981, *1,* 221-238.
Siegel, L.M., Attkisson, C.C., & Cohn, I.H. Mental health needs assessment: Strategies and techniques. In W.A. Hargreanes & C.C. Attkisson (Eds.), *Resource materials for community mental health program evaluation.* Rockville, Maryland: National Institute of Mental Health, 1977.
Warheit, George J. The use of field surveys to estimate health needs in the general population. In R.A. Bell, M. Sundel, J. Aponte, & S.A. Murell (Eds.), *Needs assessment in health and human service.* Louisville: University of Louisville, 1976.
Watzlawick, P., Weakland, J., & Fisch, R. *Change: Principles of problem formation and problem resolution.* New York: Norton, 1974.
Weimer, W. *Notes on the methodology of scientific research.* New York: Wiley, 1979.
Zuñiga, R. The experimenting society and radical social reform. *American Psychologist,* 1975, *30,* 99-115.

A Model for Monitoring Changes in Drug Use and Treatment Entry

Eugenie Walsh Flaherty
Lynne Kotranski
Elaine Fox

ABSTRACT. A model developed for use by multijurisdiction systems in monitoring and anticipating changes in drug use and treatment entry was tested in the Philadelphia system; the process of implementing the model and illustrative products are described. The model integrates data obtained from multiple archival sources and interviews with drug users by means of the census tract; other geographic units can be used. Archival data sources considered include treatment programs, hospital emergency rooms, private physicians, criminal justice agencies, public health systems and schools. Sample products address the relationship of socio-environmental variables to drug use and treatment, the geographic distribution of drug activities, and trends in heroin and polydrug use.

In 1976 and 1977 Philadelphia drug treatment programs experienced a sharp drop in the number of opiate-abusers seeking treatment entry. By late summer of 1977 it was clear that this was neither a seasonal trend nor a trend limited to a single indicator. Both treatment admissions and readmissions declined from the last quarter of 1976 to the last quarter of 1977 by 55% and cases coming into hospital emergency rooms for treatment of heroin, morphine, or methadone problems fell sharply in the last quarter of 1976. Even

Work on this article was supported by the National Institute on Drug Abuse (H82DA02066). The authors thank DeWitt Kay and Christopher D'Amanda for their extensive assistance on the work described in this article, and two anonymous reviewers for their incisive comments. The views expressed are the authors' and do not necessarily represent the views of the National Institute on Drug Abuse. Requests for reprints should be sent to the second author at the Philadelphia Health Management Corporation, 841 Chestnut St., Philadelphia, PA 19107.

89

monthly urinalysis data for clients in treatment showed fewer positive tests for opiates. Philadelphia police, in the first half of 1977, picked up 32% fewer cases requiring drug detoxification and made fewer arrests for both the sale and manufacture of heroin and for drug-related property crimes. Furthermore, this reduction in heroin activity and treatment demand was occurring simultaneously in most urban areas nationwide, including Boston, New York, San Francisco, and Miami (D'Amanda, 1978).

The phenomenon of declining admissions, labeled *demand reduction* (Bencivengo, 1978), revealed the inability of urban treatment systems to plan for changes in heroin activity and treatment demand and thus to prevent consequent problems. In retrospect, there were early indicators, but city planners did not have available to them any means of integrating and comparing different data sources in order to understand and perhaps prevent or limit the widespread nature of the decline reflected in these indicators. Lack of such a system stimulated the project described in this paper. The project goal was to develop and test a model which cities can use to anticipate changes in drug use and in treatment demand and to prevent the undesired consequences of those changes.

In selecting methods, there were a number of important considerations. Most important was a capacity for analysis of small intra-city geographic units appropriate for planning by individual cities. In Philadelphia, census tracts were used because most data sources were available or could be aggregated by tracts and because this unit was judged useful for planning. (Other units potentially useful to cities are voting wards, planning districts, block groups, boroughs, and neighborhood sectors.) Second, in recognition of increased polydrug use, access to use of both heroin and other drugs (synthetic opiates, sedatives, stimulants, hallucinogens, and tranquilizers) was to be monitored. Third, the data had to be timely and low cost in order to encourage ongoing use by cities in tracking drug changes. Fourth, it had to be possible to integrate into a city treatment system's routine monitoring procedures. Finally, there were to be multiple methods and data sources, as triangulation was judged essential in monitoring phenomena like drug use and treatment entry, where what little we know suggests multiple correlates (Leserman, 1977; Schlenger & Greenberg, 1980).

Three categories of data were selected to satisfy these concerns:

1. Social area analysis of data relevant to susceptibility to social

problems in order to examine the association between socio-environmental characteristics and other social problems (e.g., mental health, sudden infant death) and drug use.

2. Archival data which are directly associated with drug treatment or drug use. Such archival data include police, schools, treatment programs and public health records.
3. Interview data from drug users contacted in geographic areas (census tracts) judged, through analysis of the archival data, to be of high susceptibility for drug use.

Data On Susceptibility To Social Problems

The primary task of this project was to understand two events: drug use and entry into drug treatment programs. The approach was based on the assumption that drug use is related to socio-environmental variables. Most often, the environmental variables related to these events reflect social or economic deprivation (Bordva, 1959; Boggs, 1959; Fulcomer, Pellegrini, & Lefebvre, 1981; Muhlin, Cohen, Struening, Genevie, Kaplan, & Peck, 1981) and/or minority status (Rabkin, 1979). Events found to be related to environmental variables are diverse; examples include sudden infant-death syndrome (SIDS), blackout looting, mental health status, crime, and adolescent pregnancy. Past research has also found drug use to be related to social environmental characteristics: addiction rates have been found to vary by level of income of census tracts (Brown, DuPont, & Kozel, 1973; Chein, Gerard, & Lee, 1964), housing conditions in both the census tract (Brown et al., 1973) and the city (Rutledge, Seder, & Piper, 1975), neighborhood instability (Chein et al., 1964; Dai, 1970) and the family characteristics of neighborhood residents (O'Donnell, Voss, Clayton, Slatin, & Room, 1976).

Little evidence exists, however, on the relationship of socio-environmental variables to treatment entry. A pilot study for this project suggests that treatment utilization is influenced by changes in quality and availability of heroin (Flaherty, Olsen, & Benicivengo, 1980); Green believes that heroin availability "may well be *the* major factor in determining use patterns . . ." (1977, p. 208). We may find that while relatively stable environmental characteristics (e.g., economic level, residential stability) are related to drug use, the stimulus for treatment entry lies in the fluctuating nature of drug availability. If so, treatment entry will not be found to be related to those social structural variables explored in the social area analysis; the relationship of treatment entry to drug availability can be best examined in interviews with drug users, the third category of data used in the project.

Two data sources on socio-environmental characteristics were used: the United States Census Bureau and the local Department of Public Welfare. Twenty-seven census variables were abstracted from published census reports, reflecting general demographic/ population, socio-economic, family and household, neighborhood stability, and housing characteristics. Selection of these variables was based on prior research employing social area analysis which suggested that these variables make up three factor components accounting for most of the social variability among census tracts in urban areas (Johnston, 1976; Tryon, 1955). Using cluster analysis, the three social area factor components, first found by Tryon, were identified: socio-economic independence, family status, and assimilation/ethnicity.[1] All residential census tracts in the city were assigned scores on each of the three factor components.

Two sets of data were obtained from the local Department of Public Welfare (DPW): numbers of persons receiving Aid to Families with Dependent Children (AFDC) and numbers of persons receiving general assistance (GA). The DPW office provided a printout of all data requested by census tract for 1972; these raw data were then computed as rates (per 10,000 population) for each census tract. For years after 1972, however, data were not available by tract; all analyses thus used 1972 assistance data only.

ARCHIVAL DATA SOURCES ASSOCIATED WITH TREATMENT ENTRY

There are four archival sources of data on clients receiving treatment for drug use, each of which is briefly described: city treatment programs, Veterans Administration programs, hospital emergency rooms, and private physicians.

---

[1]Each factor component was made up of several variables: *Socioeconomic Independence Factor.* Median school years completed, percent employed in professional occupations, median family income, median house value, median gross rent. *Family Status Factor.* Persons per household, percent husband-wife families with children, percent owner-occupied housing units, rooms per housing unit, percent single unit structures. *Assimilation/ Ethnicity Factor.* Percent white population, percent foreign stock, percent employed as laborers.

Client Oriented Data Acquisition Process (CODAP)

CODAP provides quarterly data for all federally funded treatment programs on client admission and discharge. CODAP's utility to city planners is limited by four characteristics: (1) a one-year delay in reporting of data; (2) lack of client locational identifiers such as zip code, census tract or address, effectively limiting analyses to the city as a whole or to individual treatment programs; (3) inaccuracy of information normally found in data required of programs by external agencies; and (4) omission of data on clients in other than federally funded programs. Fortunately, the Philadelphia drug treatment system has an alternative source of treatment data which contains client addresses, through its Central Medical Intake (CMI), a federally-funded intake and referral center for approximately half the clients entering city programs. There were no significant differences between CMI-referred clients and non-CMI clients on sex, age, primary drug, educational level, and treatment modality, although CMI-referred clients did include a higher percentage of non-whites (72.3%) than did non-CMI clients (50.6%). Judging the CMI clients sufficiently representative of the whole, and knowing that we had no other options, CMI data were used. Addresses for all clients entering CMI in 1978 were converted to census tracts.

The Veterans Administration (VA)

The VA provided a list of clients by address for the years 1976 to 1979; these addresses were converted to census tracts. This data source is especially important because the VA treats a higher percentage of white clients and clients with advanced education than city programs (McLellan, O'Brien, Luborsky, & Woody, 1981). Accordingly, use of the two sets of data (VA and CMI) together increases the representativeness of the treatment sample.

Drug Abuse Warning Network (DAWN)

Hospital emergency rooms provide data on drug users receiving treatment for drug crises; these data are of special interest because they include drug users who tend not to enter traditional drug rehabilitation programs (e.g., women, the middle-class, polydrug users), as well as those whose appearances at an emergency room constitute a warning signal for a new and potentially dangerous drug or a change in quality of a known drug (National Institute on Drug Abuse/Drug Enforcement Agency, 1979). Emergency room data on non-fatal drug emergencies are collected by the Drug Abuse Warning Network (DAWN) from a sample of volunteer non-federal hospitals with emergency rooms open 24 hours a day and with at least 1,000 visits per year of any type. DAWN drug use data are reported by drug mentions, not by individual; thus an individual with an overdose of two drugs will be recorded as two separate drug mentions. As hospital location, rather than the patient's place of residence, is recorded, the actual number of individuals involved in the drug mentions or where they live cannot be determined. Thus, although DAWN's value as an early warning signal to cities is high, the data have limited utility for planning by geographic units within urban areas. Accordingly, we decided not to include DAWN data in the project.

National Disease and Therapeutic Index (NDTI)

The National Disease and Therapeutic Index (NDTI) maintains a national panel of 1,500 physicians who report case history information four times a year on patients seen during a 48-hour period. Among many items reported are drug prescriptions, including form and dosage, and diagnosis.[2] While these data may be especially useful in studying drug use among women (who receive more than two-thirds of all the prescriptions for Valium and Librium; Porpora, 1981) they are available only on the basis of nine national regions. The size of the geographic unit makes these data useless for intracity planning.

ARCHIVAL DATA SOURCES ASSOCIATED WITH DRUG USE

The data sources discussed above provide information only about drug users who avail themselves of treatment; an assumption is required that service users are not different from nonusers on key variables. Suspecting that this assumption was not acceptable for drug use, serious consideration was given to data sources providing

---

[2]The National Drug and Therapeutic Index (NDTI) contains proprietary information belonging to IMS America, LTD., Ambler, Pennsylvania.

information on drug users other than those entering treatment. Three such sources were considered: the criminal justice, public health, and school systems.

Criminal Justice Data

Two types of criminal justice data are available. Local police departments can usually provide drug law violation breakdowns for drug-related offenses and arrests, for arrests related to the sale and manufacture of heroin, and for Type I crimes (homicide, assaults, burglary, robbery, rape, auto theft, and larceny). Geographic units for analysis will vary; in Philadelphia the data are available by police sectors, which are smaller than census tracts. Another set of criminal justice data is available from the Federal Bureau of Investigation (FBI), which reports data annually on Type I crimes and on drug law violations on the city, county and state level; these data may not be available by census tract. We chose to use local police records, reasoning that FBI data would be redundant and perhaps unavailable in intra-city geographic units. Data on drug-related offenses and arrests and Type I crimes were obtained after developing a mapping program that converted police sector boundaries to census tract demarcations.

Public Health Data

Public health data relevant to drug use can be obtained from municipal departments of public health and Medical Examiner Offices which, respectively, supply information on deaths due to hepatitis and on drug-related deaths. Deaths due to hepatitis are usually too sparse to be useful to a within-city study; less than five were recorded in Philadelphia in 1978. Accessibility and information collected will vary by City Medical Examiner Departments, but records usually include address where the body was found, which can be converted to census tract. For project purposes, we extracted from Philadelphia Medical Examiner files information on address, date of death, and drug type (heroin, other opiates, and other drugs) for all drug-related deaths.

School Data

Information on school drug use is highly desirable for planning. Because the time lag between first use of heroin and first treatment entry is fairly well understood, at least for urban, low-income, black youths, data on school drug use can be used to prevent subsequent drug use and to predict later treatment demand (Brunswick, 1979; Glenn & Richards, 1974; Lukoff, 1976; Johnston, Abbey, Scheble, & Weitman, 1972). Philadelphia public school records contain two types of information on school drug use: counselor files and police reports. Counselor files were unavailable to the project for reasons of confidentiality and in any case would have been too time-consuming to use. Police reports were available, but permission was given only for use of school address, not student address. Because the majority of students live relatively near their school, school addresses were judged to be adequate; these addresses were extracted, along with drug type, and converted to census tract.

Unfortunately, review of the school data suggested significant under-reporting and biases in reporting. Ninety-five percent of the incidents reported were for marijuana use, and proportionately fewer drug incidents were reported from inner-city schools in the poorest neighborhoods, neighborhoods which had copping or drug dealing areas near the schools. The questionable validity of the school data led to a decision not to use them in the analyses.

DATA ON "STREET" DRUG USE

We employed three sources to obtain information about street drug use and the street drug user (that is, the user who is not currently in contact with an institution): Drug Enforcement Administration (DEA) agents, treatment program staff, and interviewers working on the street and in treatment programs. The last source violated two of the desired characteristics of the model, ready data availability and minimal cost, yet was judged essential to gain information on non-institutional drug users. Use of interviews could be omitted without interfering with the remaining model methods.

DEA Agents

DEA agents routinely purchase heroin, cocaine and methamphetamines in urban copping areas, locations where "corner level" dealers (the lowest level in the dealing hierarchy) sell drugs. These agents are thus quite knowledgeable about geographic patterns of drug dealing. Eighty-six individual copping areas were identified by the agents, and the presence or absence of a copping area was then coded for each census tract.

Treatment Program Staff

Treatment program staff, in a special exercise created for the project, "mapped" severity of use of heroin, synthetic opiates, and amphetamines separately for each census tract in the city. Nine staff members met in groups of three to work with a large city census tract map. The groups worked with one drug at a time, until a consensus was reached about the severity of drug activity in each tract. Individual differences in familiarity with census tracts were dealt with by the group, which usually asked the more familiar member to justify his rating by describing tract activity. As census tracts were dealt with, colors corresponding to severity codes were filled in so the group could see the map evolve. When completed, the groups' responses were numerically coded for each census tract using a four-point scale. It is important to note that the mapping exercise is a difficult task for both group leader and participant: Philadelphia has three hundred and sixty-four census tracts, and as much as possible, participants were prevented from grouping tracts together. The time-consuming exercise requires skilled group leaders and participants who appreciate the project's purpose.

Ethnographic Interviewers

Use of ethnographic interviewers in drug abuse research is not unique to this project: New York, Chicago, Philadelphia, and San Francisco have used highly trained ethnographers in a variety of efforts (McCall & Simmons, 1969), including routine monitoring of the drug scene in high-risk areas of the city, a one-time study of the effects of drug use among Hispanic families, a study of amphetamine users and diet-pill doctors, and a one-time study, requested by a city councilman, of reported abuse by adolescents of "loony balloony," tubes of plastic cement blown through a straw into a balloon (Johnson & Lipton, 1980). While employment of professional ethnographers would be productive for all cities, such employment is also costly, requires very careful selection of ethnographic staff, and assumes supervisors in the treatment system trained in ethnography.

In this project we developed an interview instrument and procedures which included some important qualities of ethnographic data collection, but avoided the limitations listed above. Briefly, nine interviewers were selected who were experienced with drug users but not highly experienced in research interviewing. The interviewers received intensive training in the use of a standardized interview consisting of both closed- and open-ended questions (see Fox, Kotranski, & Flaherty, 1982, for a detailed description of this training). Respondents included drug users entering treatment (although not necessarily for the first time), (n = 93), and "street" drug users not currently in treatment (n = 300).

The "street" respondents were selected from census tracts shown to be highest in drug use through analysis of the archival data (see below). The interviewers worked in assigned census tracts and selected drug-using respondents who "hung out" or lived in those census tracts. Interviews took place in bars, "open houses," copping areas, parks, and on street corners. Treatment programs were selected to yield respondents demographically representative of the high drug use census tracts.

Selection of high drug use census tracts was based on three indices: location of one or more copping areas in a census tract, severity ratings of heroin use in census tracts obtained from the mapping exercise, and population-adjusted drug-related death rates for each census tract. All tracts containing at least one copping area and a mapping exercise rating of "major" or "severe" for heroin use were selected. These tracts were then ranked by drug-related deaths and a number of respondents proportionate to the tract's population, but not less than five, was assigned to each tract.

This selection process yielded 28 tracts which were predominantly nonwhite and low-income. Because a pilot study (Flaherty et al., 1980) and ethnographic work being conducted in other cities suggested that much polydrug activity was occurring in white and working-class neighborhoods as well, four additional census tracts were added. Four clusters of tracts in predominantly white working-class neighborhoods containing at least one copping area were identified, and the tract with the highest heroin severity rating and rate of drug-related deaths was selected from each cluster.

All study respondents met two inclusion criteria: they had to be eighteen or over and had to have used heroin at least once during the twelve-month period prior to the interview. The latter criterion avoided limiting the sample to users who predominantly used heroin, and yet assured that all respondents had been exposed to heroin. Respondents could conceivably not be using any drug at the time of the interview (this was rare) or be using many drugs, including heroin (this was most common).

The one-hour length of the interview was too long for routine city use, but the interview is made up of separate sections which can be employed independently to address particular needs. The interview had four major sections: respondent's drug use and treatment history, respondent's life style as it relates to drug use, perceptions of friends' drug use, and opinions about causes of recent changes in drug use and treatment entry. Six categories of drugs were dealt with in each section: heroin, synthetic opiates, sedative hypnotics, stimulants, hallucinogens, and tranquilizers. The interviews were tape-recorded, and the interviewer subsequently listened to the tape to augment notes on the questionnaire form. Although most of the questionnaire was ready for keypunching when handed in, certain sections of the tapes were transcribed verbatim in order to increase understanding of the respondents' responses.

SAMPLE QUESTIONS AND FINDINGS
FROM THE PHILADELPHIA DEMONSTRATION

In this section we demonstrate the utility of this approach by posing questions typically asked about urban drug use and using the data collected in Philadelphia to answer them. These questions are by no means the only ones which can be answered through this approach; they were selected to demonstrate the variation in information needs met by the approach. All analyses utilizing archival data used the census tract as their unit of analysis.

Are Socio-Environmental Variables Related to Drug Use?

As discussed earlier, selected social and health problems, such as juvenile delinquency (Bordva, 1959), sudden infant death (Fulcomer et al., 1981), adolescent pregnancy (Flaherty, Marecek, Olsen, & Wilcove, 1982), and even blackout looting (Muhlin et al., 1981), are associated with an environment of social and/or economic deprivation and other social problems. Is drug use as well? Three variables in the data set may reflect social problems (measured by homicide rates, suicide rates, public assistance rates), whereas the three factor components identified through social area analysis of census variables—socioeconomic independence (S), family status (F), and assimilation/ethnicity (A)—are global measures of the social environment. All three census factors exhibited relatively high correlations with homicides (r = .44, -.27, and -.70 with S, F, and A respectively) and with public assistance rates (r = .55, -.29, and .78 with S, F, and A respectively) and somewhat lower correlations with suicides (r = .21, .16, .13 with S, F, A). Suicides seem to be somewhat independent of the other variables, having non-significant relationships with public assistance rates (r = .04) and homicides (r = .04).

Do these social area factors explain any variance in drug use or treatment utilization? Five indicators of drug use were available in the data set: drug-related death rates, copping area locations, and three "mappings" of severity of use by treatment staff, for heroin, synthetic opiates and amphetamines. Two indicators of treatment utilization were used: Veterans Administration (VA) admissions for 1976-79 and Central Medical Intake (CMI) admissions for 1978. Using multiple regression techniques, the combined and relative (independent) effects of the three social area factors (socioeconomic independence, family status, and assimilation/ethnicity) in predicting drug use and treatment utilization were examined (Table 1).

The three social area factors appear to explain a much greater proportion of the variance in drug use than in treatment utilization. Thirty-five to fifty-four percent of the variance in all indicators of drug use, with the exception of copping areas, is explained, with all three environmental factors having significant effects. In comparison, only sixteen and twenty percent of the variance in CMI and VA admissions, respectively, is explained. The social area factors are most successful in predicting heroin use (R^2 = .54), and least successful in predicting the presence of copping areas (R^2 = .17) and CMI admissions (R^2 = .16).

These data suggest qualitative differences in the correlates, and probably the underlying mechanisms, accounting for drug use and treatment utilization. Prior research, discussed above, also supports relationships between drug use and socio-environmental factors. What, then, influences treatment utilization? Evidence supports the "burning-out" thesis, whereby older heroin addicts (generally users of at least ten years) stop using heroin spontaneously (Stephens & Cottrell, 1972; Winick, 1965), but this phenomenon does not explain treatment utilization measured in the aggregate nor the phenomenon of demand reduction which stimulated this study. A

Table 1

Regression Analysis of Drug Use and Treatment Utilization Indicators on Social Area Factors (Philadelphia census tracts, n=347)

| Indicators | Social Area Factors Standardized Regression Coefficients | | | | |
	Socioeconomic Independence	Family Status	Assimilation/ ethnicity	R	R^2
Drug Use:					
Drug-related death rates (1970-78)	-.208***	-.215***	-.469***	.67	.45
Severity ratings of heroin use	-.292***	-.156***	-.499***	.74	.54
Severity ratings of synthetic opiate use	-.298***	-.145***	-.395***	.64	.41
Severity ratings of amphetamine use	-.236***	.116**	-.441***	.59	.35
Presence of copping area [a]	-.079	-.181***	-.291***	.41	.17
Treatment Utilization:					
Veteran's Administration Admissions	-.103*	-.022	.376***	.44	.20
Central Medical Intake Admissions	-.283***	-.155***	-.117**	.40	.16

[a] Dummy variable coded (1=presence of copping area; 0=absence of copping area)

* $p < .05$
** $p < .01$
*** $p < .001$

101

pilot study conducted towards the end of the course of demand reduction suggested that at that time (spring of 1978) the decline in treatment utilization was associated with decreased quality and availability of heroin and increased polydrug use (Flaherty et al., 1980). However, the interviews conducted in this project, during the spring and summer of 1981, suggest that heroin availability was not a problem then; 90.2% of the respondents said they had no trouble obtaining heroin, although 42.2% did complain that the heroin was weaker than it had been a year before. During this time treatment utilization for heroin was actually rising (Coordinating Office of Drug & Alcohol Abuse, 1981). Respondents who were entering treatment at the time of the interview indicated that they entered treatment because of a need to change their lifestyle (97.8%), to bring their habit down and "cool out" (92.7%), to improve their health (92.7%), to get or hold a job (81.7%), to improve family relationships (78.5%), and because they were tired of "being strung out and ripped off" (77.4%). Only 46.2% cited poor drug quality as a motive.

These data suggest that when there is a marked decline in heroin availability and quality treatment utilization decreases as well, since physiological addiction is not strong and can be dealt with either through substitution of other drugs or by cessation on one's own. When heroin availability and quality are not a problem, as seems to have been the case in 1981, the interview data suggest that those who enter treatment do so for a variety of reasons which can be labeled "lifestyle improvement." The individual's motive to improve his lifestyle is probably not a direct function of socio-demographic environmental variables as measured on an area basis (census tract).

How Are Drug Activities Distributed Across the City?

Because geographic mapping of indicators is useful to city planners and system administrators, to whom visually arrayed distributions may be more meaningful than use of statistical prediction techniques, we developed a mapping capability for displaying the data. This technique is illustrated in Figures 1 and 2 which show the treatment staff's ratings of heroin use and CMI admissions for 1978. Maps have also been prepared to illustrate the geographic distributions of staff ratings of synthetic opiate and amphetamine use severity, copping areas, drug-related deaths and VA admissions.

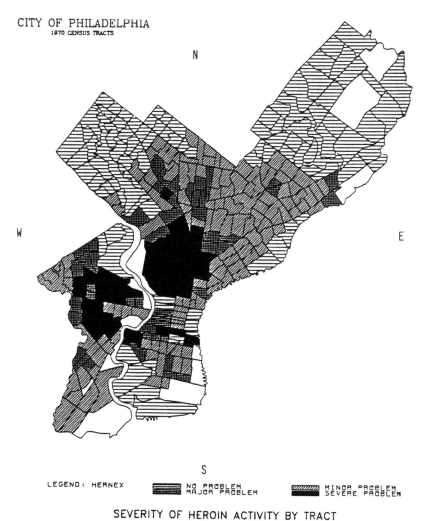

CITY OF PHILADELPHIA
1970 CENSUS TRACTS

N

W

E

S

LEGEND: HERNEX

NO PROBLEM
MAJOR PROBLEM

MINOR PROBLEM
SEVERE PROBLEM

SEVERITY OF HEROIN ACTIVITY BY TRACT
(NEXUS RATINGS)

Do Heroin Users Also Use Other Drugs; and If So, Which Ones? Is the Degree of Heroin Use Changing?

Approximately two-thirds of the respondents interviewed reported using heroin at least once a day (66.2%, $n = 260$), while one-third used heroin less than daily (33.8%, $n = 133$). Females (61.0%) were almost as likely as males (67.4%) to report using

CITY OF PHILADELPHIA
1970 CENSUS TRACTS

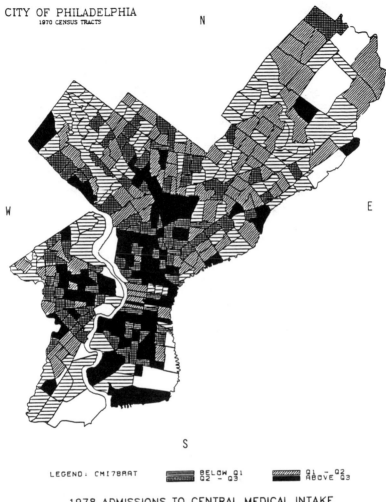

LEGEND: CMI78RRT   BELOW Q1 / Q2 - Q3   Q1 - Q2 / ABOVE Q3

1978 ADMISSIONS TO CENTRAL MEDICAL INTAKE
(PER 10,000 POPULATION)

heroin every day. Of those respondents who used heroin less than daily, one-third had not used any heroin in the past month (although they had in the past year), one-third reported using heroin once in the past month, and one-third had used it at least weekly during the past month.

Do respondents in this sample of heroin users use other drugs as well? At least 80 percent of all respondents reported using synthetic opiates, stimulants and tranquilizers in the past year, and most of these had used those drugs in the past month. Only hallucinogens appeared relatively unpopular; twenty-nine percent of the respondents had used a hallucinogen in the last year, and only 60.0% of these (*n* = 69) (or 17.5% of the total sample) used them in the past month.

Respondents who used heroin at least once a day did not seem very different from those who used it less frequently in terms of the other drugs they used. Generally, most respondents of both types seemed to use other drugs often, suggesting that polydrug use represents the norm rather than the exception among heroin users. The most frequently used drugs in the various categories are as follows:

> *Synthetic opiates*—codeine, methadone, Talwin and Benadryl (also known as "soup"), and Ritalin and Talwin ("Ritz and Ts").
> *Sedative hypnotics*—tuinals, seconal, quaaludes, and doriden.
> *Stimulants*—cocaine and methedrine ("speed").
> *Hallucinogens*—PCP ("angel dust"), LSD, and THC.
> *Tranquilizers*—valium and librium.

Despite prevalent polydrug use, respondents were not necessarily using less heroin than they had a year ago. Approximately half (48.3%) reported using less, but one-third (33.0%) reported using more and 18.7 percent reported using the same amount.

DISCUSSION

A model has been proposed and tested for use in anticipating changes in drug use and treatment entry. The model makes use of multiple methods and data sources, integrated by means of a common geographic unit. Its application is thus useful for any drug rehabilitation system with jurisdiction over a relatively large area divisible into units of a size useful for planning.

Current and accurate knowledge of drug use is essential for planning to prevent both increased drug use and attendant medical problems as well as unanticipated treatment demand. As the findings in this project suggest, reliance on a single indicator to reflect drug use changes can be very misleading and result in inappropriate preven-

Table 2

Use of Drugs Other than Heroin by Daily and Occasional Heroin Users

Frequency of use during past month [a]	Daily Heroin Users (N=260)		Occasional Heroin Users (N=133)		All Users (N=393)	
	N	%	N	%	N	%
Synthetic Opiates:						
not at all	27	11.5	22	18.3	49	13.8
monthly/weekly	115	48.9	51	42.5	166	46.8
daily	93	39.6	47	39.2	140	39.4
total	235	90.4[b]	120	90.2[b]	355	90.3[b]
Sedative Hypnotics:						
not at all	20	12.0	19	21.1	39	15.2
monthly/weekly	100	60.0	56	62.2	156	60.7
daily	47	28.0	15	16.7	62	24.1
total	167	64.2[b]	90	67.7[b]	257	65.5[b]
Stimulants:						
not at all	14	17.0	16	12.7	30	8.2
monthly/weekly	169	70.7	79	62.7	248	68.0
daily	56	23.4	31	24.6	87	23.8
total	239	91.9[b]	126	94.8[b]	365	92.9[b]
Hallucinogens:						
not at all	18	27.7	27	55.1	45	39.5
monthly/weekly	44	67.7	21	42.9	65	57.0
daily	3	4.6[b]	1	2.0	4	3.5
total	65	25.0[b]	49	36.8[b]	114	29.0[b]
Tranquilizers:						
not at all	17	8.1	16	13.4	33	10.0
monthly/weekly	115	54.8	67	56.3	182	55.3
daily	78	37.1	36	30.3	114	34.7
total	210	80.8[b]	119	89.5[b]	329	83.7[b]

[a] This question was asked only of those who had used the given drug within the past year; thus the totals differ for each drug.
[b] This figure represents the percentage of all column respondents (e.g., N=260, 133, or 393) who reported using the drug within the past year.

tative actions. Our lack of knowledge about the correlates of drug use and treatment entry requires an approach that integrates multiple indicators.

To date the indicator most frequently used for planning is the degree and nature of utilization of treatment programs. However, many drug users do not use treatment programs, especially as polydrug use increases, and when they do use them, it is only after a lengthy period of drug use. Current knowledge of drug use would allow drug rehabilitation systems to prevent increased use of particularly dangerous drugs, perhaps through public education through the media, before users overdose or use long enough to desire treatment. Furthermore, current knowledge would assist systems to put increased and more appropriate resources into preventative actions as opposed to "after-the-fact" treatment. This model can assist drug systems to focus on earlier stages of drug use and to design efforts directed towards these earlier stages, thus preventing or at least limiting subsequent stages.

REFERENCES

Bencivengo, M. *Observations on reduced treatment-seeking among urban opiate abusers.* Paper presented to the Public Policy Section of the National Drug Abuse Conference, Seattle, Washington, April 1978.

Boggs, S.L. Urban crime patterns. *American Sociological Review*, 1959, *30*, 899-908.

Bordva, D.S. Juvenile delinquency and crime. *Social Problems*, 1959, *6*, 230-238.

Brown, B.S., DuPont, R.L., & Kozel, N.J. Heroin addiction in the city of Washington. *Drug Forum*, 1973, *2*(2), 187-190.

Brunswick, A. Black youths and drug-use behavior. In G. Beschner & A. Friedman (Eds.), *Youth drug abuse.* Lexington, Massachusetts: D.C. Heath, 1979.

Chein, I., Gerard, D.L., & Lee, R.S. *The road to h: Narcotics, delinquency, and social policy.* New York: Basic Books, 1964.

Coordinating Office of Drug and Alcohol Abuse Problems. *Uniform data collection system annual report.* City of Philadelphia Department of Public Health, 1981.

Dai, B. *Opium addiction in Chicago.* Montclair, New Jersey: Patterson Smith, 1970.

D'Amanda, C. *Philadelphia city report to community correspondents' group.* City of Philadelphia, Coordinating Office of Drug and Alcohol Abuse Problems, January 1978.

Flaherty, E.W., Marecek, J.S., Olsen, K., & Wilcove, G. *Psychological factors associated with fertility regulation among adolescents.* Final Report, contract No. 1N01-HD-82833, National Institute of Child Health and Human Development, Rockville, MD, January 1982.

Flaherty, E.W., Olsen, K., & Bencivengo, M. Predicting changes in drug use and treatment entry for local programs: A case study. *American Journal of Drug and Alcohol Abuse,* 1980, *7*(1), 31-48.

Fox, E., Kotranski, L., & Flaherty, E.W. *The use of indigenous field interviewers for semi-ethnographic survey research on urban drug abusers.* Paper presented at the annual meetings of the Eastern Sociological Society, Philadelphia, PA, March 1982.

Fulcomer, M.C., Pellegrini, S.G., & Lefebvre, L.C. Demographic and health-related predictors of the incidence of sudden infant death. *Evaluation and Program Planning,* 1981, *4*(1), 43-56.

Glenn, W.A., & Richards, L.G. *Recent surveys of nonmedical drug use: A compendium of abstracts.* Rockville, MD: National Institute on Drug Abuse, 1974.

Greene, M.H. Applications of indicator data: Discussions. In L. Richards & L. Blevens (Eds.), *The epidemiology of drug abuse* (NIDA Research Monograph Series 10). Washington, D.C.: U.S. Government Printing Office, 1977.

Johnson, B.D., & Lipton, D.S. Creative tensions: Issues in utilizing ethnographic research within a Single State Agency. In L. Atkins & G. Beschner (Eds.), *Ethnography: A research tool for policymakers in the drug and alcohol fields* (DHHS Publication No. (ADM) 80-946). Washington, D.C.: U.S. Government Printing Office, 1980.

Johnston, K.G., Abbey, H., Scheble, R., & Weitman, M. Survey of adolescent drug use: Social and environmental factors. *American Journal of Public Health,* 1972, 164-166.

Johnston, R.J. Residential area characteristics: Research methods for identifying urban sub-area analysis and factorial ecology. In D. Herbert & R. Johnston (Eds), *Social areas in cities: Special processes and forms.* New York: John Wiley & Sons, 1976.

Leserman, J. *Identification of variables associated with the prevalence of heroin use.* Research Triangle Park, North Carolina: Research Triangle Institute, 1977.

Lukoff, I.F. Consequences of use: Heroin and other narcotics. In J.D. Rittenhouse (Ed.), *The epidemiology of heroin and other narcotics.* Menlo Park, California: Stanford Research Institute, 1976.

McCall, G.S., & Simmons, J.L. *Issues in participant observation: A text and reader.* Reading, Maine: Addison-Wesley, 1969.

McLellan, A.T., O'Brien, C.P., Luborsky, L., & Woody, G.E. Certain types of substance abuse patients do better in certain kinds of treatment. In *Problems of drug dependence* (National Institute on Drug Abuse Research Monograph 34). Washington, D.C.: U.S. Government Printing Office, 1981.

Muhlin, G.L., Cohen, P., Struening, E.L., Genevie, L.E., Kaplan, S.R., & Peck, H.B. Behavioral epidemiology and social area analysis: The study of blackout looting. *Evaluation and Program Planning,* 1981, *4*(1), 35-42.

National Institute on Drug Abuse/Drug Enforcement Agency. *Project DAWN annual report.* Ambler, Pennsylvania: IMS America, LTD., 1979.

O'Donnell, J.A., Voss, H.L., Clayton, R.R., Slatin, G.T., & Room, R.G. *Young men and drugs: A nationwide survey* (NIDA Research Monograph 5). National Institute on Drug Abuse, Rockville, MD, 1976.

Porpora, D. *Physician prescriptions for tranquilizers and tranquilizer abuse.* Paper presented at the annual meetings of the Eastern Sociological Society, Philadelphia, PA, March 1982.

Rabkin, J.G. Ethnic density and psychiatric hospitalization: Hazards of minority status. *American Journal of Psychiatry,* 1979, *136,* 1562-1566.

Rutledge, J., Seder, P., & Piper, R. *Opiate addiction and urban conditions: A social indicator analysis.* National League of Cities, U.S. Conference of Mayors, Washington, D.C., 1975.

Schlenger, W.E., & Greenberg, S.W. Characteristics of cities and their relationship to heroin use: An analysis of heroin use correlates in metropolitan areas. *International Journal of the Addictions,* 1980, *15*(8), 1141-1168.

Stephens, R.C., & Cottrell, E.A. A follow-up study of 200 narcotic addicts committed for treatment under the Narcotic Rehabilitation Act (NARA). *British Journal of Addiction,* 1972, *67,* 45-53.

Tryon, R.C. *Identification of social areas by cluster analysis.* Stanford: Stanford University Press, 1955.

Winick, C. Epidemiology of narcotics use. In D. Wilner & G. Kassenbaum (Eds.), *Narcotics.* New York: McGraw-Hill, 1965.

Primary Prevention for Children:
A Framework
for the Assessment of Need

Robert D. Felner
Mark S. Aber

ABSTRACT. This paper discusses the role of needs assessment procedures in the development of effective primary prevention strategies for children and youth. A number of techniques which may be employed in the assessment of need for such services are presented and their strengths and limitations for such application are discussed. Particular problems for needs assessment planning and implementation stemming from differences in the goals and objectives of preventive, as opposed to more traditional mental health services for children, are elaborated and possible strategies for their resolution suggested.

Programs designed to prevent emotional disturbance have been increasingly accorded a position of central importance in the mental health service delivery system (President's Commission Report on Mental Health, 1978). While programs included under the broad rubric of prevention at times include efforts targeted at individuals already displaying psychological maladaptation (e.g., secondary prevention) it is with that group of programs which have been labeled ''primary prevention'' which this paper is concerned. Numer-

Preparation of this paper was in part supported by Grant DAR 80-11001 from the National Science Foundation. Appreciation is due to Alex Zautra for his helpful comments on earlier drafts.

Requests for reprints should be sent to Robert D. Felner, Department of Psychology, Auburn University, Auburn, AL 36849.

ous authors have bemoaned the lack of a stringent definition for primary prevention as an impediment to the development of a sound knowledge base upon which to build effective programs (Cowen, 1980; Price, Bader, & Ketterer, 1980). Generally, however, the key goals of primary prevention programs may be broadly subsumed under either: (1) the reduction of new cases of psychological disorder, and/or (2) the promotion of health and building of competence as protection against dysfunction (Cowen, 1980).

A perhaps more difficult problem than agreeing on a definition confronts those concerned with developing primary prevention programs. That is, once we decide what it is, how do we do it? The need for a more clearly articulated, shared, and rigorously pursued methodology has been pointed to as essential to achieving the goal of developing effective primary prevention programs (Price et al., 1980). Toward this end, attention to issues such as target population identification, program structure and design, and careful evaluation is clearly critical. However, there is a key prior step in the development of any human service program. This step is the careful definition and assessment of community need for the program (Cox, Carmichael, & Dightman, 1979). Baker (1974) has gone so far as to argue that no rational human service system can be created in the absence of such need assessment and definition.

Primary prevention efforts may be targeted to a wide array of populations, and it is beyond the scope of this work to address the specific issues involved in needs assessment procedures applicable to the full range of potential target populations. Rather, we will endeavor to address needs assessment procedures as they relate to a group which has frequently been singled out as the target group of "choice" for preventive efforts—children. Cowen (1980) and others (Felner, Farber, & Primavera, 1980) have argued that when decisions must be made as to where to target limited mental health financial and human resources, children are a group for whom the potential exists for obtaining maximal return on resource expenditures. In the following pages we will first discuss some of the current conceptions of needs assessment and strategies for collecting data on need in light of our focus on primary prevention programs for children. Following that we will elaborate some of the key issues and problems which confront human service professionals and agencies concerned with the assessment of children's mental health needs for the planning of such programming.

CONCEPTUALIZATION AND STRATEGIES

Definitions of what constitutes a "need" toward which to target human service programs vary in both their inclusiveness and specificity. How the need to be assessed is defined has limiting and shaping implications both for the strategies adopted to perform the needs assessment and also for the nature of the interventions which follow. Similarly, needs assessment strategies employed may subtlely, or not so subtlely, serve to define and limit our understanding of what, in fact, constitutes a need for mental health services.

Due to having their "roots" in more traditional views of service delivery, many of the definitions and indicators of needs employed by human service planners require significant modification if they are to be more than marginally applicable to the concerns of primary prevention. For example, Nguyen, Attkisson, and Bottino (1976) have defined need in this way: "An unmet need is said to exist when a problem in living, a dysfunctional somatic or psychological state or an undesirable social process is recognized, for which a satisfactory solution requires a major mobilization of additional resources and/or a major reallocation of existing resources" (p. 42). Such a definition clearly poses problems for primary prevention, particularly in its reflection of the emphasis of most human service programs on providing after-the-fact services. Only the targeting of "an undesirable social process" in the above definition allows for addressing programs to some individuals who are not already showing problems. A definition of needs assessment which is perhaps better suited for prevention activities is provided by Kamis who states, "Need assessment is an activity which provides a description and/or measure of either the relative or the absolute needs of people, living in a defined area for: (1) enhancement of a facet that is lacking in the residents' lives; (2) specific services, interventions, or programs; (3) prevention of problems that will require intervention" (1979, p. 7).

Certainly Kamis' approach more adequately allows for prevention activities than does that of Nguyen et al. (1976). However, while the Kamis approach broadens the scope of issues that needs assessment may be targeted toward, so too does it decrease the specificity and clarity of the definition of what actually constitutes a need and how it is identified. Understanding the differences between

these definitions may be helpful for illuminating one of the key difficulties in conceptualizing the need for primary prevention services for children or other groups.

The concept of need from a primary prevention standpoint is
quite different from that which results from more traditional views.
From the latter perspective a need may be said to be present when an
individual demonstrates some clearly identifiable adaptive difficul-
ty. Such is not the case for primary prevention. Indeed, when such
adaptive difficulties are present it is by definition too late for
primary prevention. We are confronted then with the task of identifying and defining need in such a way that allows for its assessment
when no adaptive problems are yet manifest in the target individuals. It is critical that planners of preventive services recognize
this issue and understand that what constitutes evidence of need for
service will, for such programs, be quite different than that which
would support the planning of other mental health services. Clear
indices of need for traditional programming may be unsuitable or
only indirectly applicable for such purposes with preventive programming. An example may help here.

In a recent paper, Felner, Norton, Cowen and Farber (1981)
report on the development of a school based prevention program for
children experiencing potentially risk predisposing life events. A
central concern raised about the implementation of this project by
some school personnel was about the need for a program for
children who "didn't display any problems." From a traditional
perspective this was, of course, a valid question as the target children were those not manifesting school adjustment problems. Certainly, it seemed to some that this program was, at best, a diversion
of resources from those children who were really "in need"—i.e.,
those with clearly identifiable difficulties. However, from a preventive perspective, to wait until dysfunctional behavior developed in
some of the target children before offering "treatment" to them
would be antithetical to the purpose of the program. Fortunately, in
this case, in-service training programs for school personnel, geared
toward educating them as to the nature and purpose of primary
prevention programs, served to help overcome this resistance to
providing service to children whose behavior did not yet appear to
need it. Nonetheless, this example illustrates the difficulties that individuals holding a more traditional orientation toward mental
health problems may have in perceiving the needs for services in the
absence of discernable behavior problems. However, as noted, to

wait for such problems to be present until attempting to justify service is contradictory to the goals of prevention.

While primary prevention's goals require a redefinition of need for service, they do not prohibit obtaining clear indicators of need to aid program planning and justification. Toward that end, let us now examine some of the more commonly discussed and utilized assessment strategies for human service programming and their potential for preventive planning.

Potentially one of the most helpful needs assessment strategies for planners of children's prevention services is that of social indicators analysis. Although not without its critics (Cochran, 1979), this approach enjoys wide acceptance among policymakers (Warheit, Buhl, & Bell, 1978) and seems particularly suitable for primary prevention planning with children. Social indicator assessment procedures are based on the idea that human service needs of a population group may be related to certain demographic, social, and economic characteristics (e.g., socioeconomic status, race, community stability) of the area in which they live (Warheit et al., 1978). Such data, derived from census records, community surveys or other sources, may be particularly helpful in identifying groups of individuals at relatively greater risk for the development of mental health problems (Cox et al., 1979). This strategy offers both the opportunity to obtain clear and quantifiable indicators of need while at the same time allowing for before-the-fact programming. Further, with groups identified as at risk by such procedures, both efforts to avoid the development of new problems as well as to enhance current functioning through programming aimed at competence building may be well justified.

Another particularly useful strategy for identifying groups with relatively greater need for preventive service is a more specific instance of social indicator analysis. A number of authors (Bloom, 1979; Dohrenwend, 1978; Felner et al., 1980; Felner, Primavera, & Cauce, 1981) have argued that preventive intervention programs should be organized around the mastery of stressful life events or transitions by individuals who experience them. The basis of this argument is that while the experience of a stressful life event places an individual at heightened risk for the development of maladaptation, services which increase their coping abilities at this time may forestall the development of such difficulties (Felner, Norton, Cowen, & Farber, 1981). For children, the potentially negative consequences of such stressful events as parental death or divorce, hospitalization, school transfer, and birth of a sibling, among others, have been well documented (Birtchnell, 1969; Felner, Ginter, Boike, & Cowen, 1981; Felner, Primavera, & Cauce, 1981; Jessner, Bloom, & Waldfogel, 1952; Legg, Sherick, & Wadland, 1974). Thus, arguments for preventive services aimed at children experiencing these or similar "risk marker" events are well supported by base rate epidemiological data, while still allowing for the targeting of programs to children not yet manifesting any adjustment difficulties.

Again, potential sources of data on the prevalence of high risk indicators and stressors may come from a combination of census tract data and carefully developed community surveys. The potential utility of these procedures has been well demonstrated in several recent studies of the impact of life stress on children (Gersten, Langner, Eisenberg, & Simcha-Fagen, 1977; Padilla, Padilla, Morales, Olmedo, & Ramirez, 1979).

The aforementioned needs identification strategies offer additional advantages over other procedures that are particularly salient for planners of children's services. This is, they require neither direct reports of perceived difficulties and/or need, nor accessing of services, either from the children themselves or individuals associated with them. Other assessment procedures such as those which employ the rate of individuals under treatment, key informants, surveys of emotional difficulties, or community forums to determine need, while certainly of some utility, have serious limitations, especially when used with children. The more general limitations of these techniques are carefully discussed elsewhere (Cox et al., 1979; Warheit et al., 1978; Zautra & Simons, 1978) and are beyond the scope of this work. However, we will briefly highlight the particular limitations which should be attended to when employing such strategies to assess the needs for preventive services for children.

Perhaps the key limitation of these approaches is that each, to some extent, depends on the children's needs being identified by others. Children typically do not seek out services on their own. Rather, they usually depend on adults to identify their needs and obtain services for them (Felner, Norton, Cowen, & Farber, 1981). Hence, if those procedures for assessing the community needs of children which have been broadly classed as "subjective" (Zautra & Simmons, 1978) are employed (e.g., key informant, community surveys or forums), planners are dependent on the individuals who are doing the actual reporting to be both sensitive and oriented to attend to the mental health needs of children who are not showing obvious behavior problems. Unfortunately, given the focus of traditional approaches and resource shortages, much of the human service system is one which is "reactive" rather than "proactive" in its orientation (Cowen, 1983), leading to a focus on immediate, pressing problems rather than on efforts to address longer term outcomes. Children who are acting-out or displaying other adjustment difficulties are troublesome not only to themselves but those around them, generally leading to identification of need for service by involved adults and a reaction on the part of the system. By contrast, children in need of preventive services generally do not yet cause any problems for the adults with whom they come into contact. The result, then, is that when subjective needs assessment procedures are employed, the needs of this latter group are almost invariably overlooked or underestimated. It should be underscored by this example that problems assigned the highest priority for services often are not, in actual fact, optimal from the standpoint of resource expenditures/return. Rather, their lofty priority may instead be a function of the reporter biases noted.

In subjective needs assessment procedures, children's needs for service may not be recognized for reasons other than the overshadowing effects of children with existing difficulties. For instance, the needs of children at risk due to stressful life circumstances may go unnoticed or unattended due to such circumstances also acting to limit the ability of salient adults to respond. Illustratively, in their discussion of the previously mentioned program for children experiencing life crises, Felner, Norton, Cowen, and Farber (1981) note "in many instances the crisis event affecting the child may also be affecting the rest of the family . . . and may lead to the parents' inability to perceive or respond to the child's needs, thus leading to the failure of many children to receive needed services" (p. 446). Similarly, while all children in an inner-city school or making the transition to high school may be seen as at risk and in need of preventive services (Felner, Primavera, & Cauce, 1981), school resources may be so overtaxed as to preclude the perception of that need until actual problems occur (Felner, Ginter, & Primavera, 1982).

The foregoing is not to imply that subjective needs assessment procedures are without value for the planning of preventive programs. Rather, the intent is to highlight some of the factors which may, at times, act to limit their utility. Attention to these issues may serve to strengthen results obtained from such procedures. For example, in employing community surveys as aids to the planning of preventive programs for children, one factor that should be reduced, in so far as possible, is the subjectivity of judgments requested of respondents. Thus, rather than asking for an appraisal of whether or not parents perceive their children as suffering from the consequences of any stressors, it may be better to present them with lists of stressors previously demonstrated as having adverse effects for children and merely asking them to indicate their presence or absence. While still allowing for some subjectivity, the latter procedure does so to a significantly lesser extent than the former.

An additional approach to needs assessment which is frequently employed is the rates-under-treatment approach in which the extent of utilization/demand for services is used as an indicator of need. This approach, however, may be plagued by differential utilization rates resulting not from true differences in need for services, but rather from such other factors as publicity, cost, availability of alternate services, and accessing problems (Zautra & Simons, 1978). Further, just as in the case of rates of dysfunction, such utilization rates are only marginally helpful in assessing needs for before-the-fact preventive services since they are after-the-fact measures. At present then, it seems that the use of "high risk marker" and social indicator analysis strategies may be the procedures of choice for those concerned with planning and developing primary preventive services for children. Certainly, as noted above and as argued by Zautra and Simons (1978), subjective assessment procedures may be a helpful adjunct to such data, particularly for getting a more fine grained look at specific need. However, if confronted by time and resource limitations, the former strategies are those which seem to be essential, particularly for preventive efforts with children.

THE DEVELOPMENT OF A STRATEGY
FOR NEEDS ASSESSMENT

In developing an overall strategy to assess children's needs for preventive services, the choice of which assessment technique to employ is not the only issue which planners of such services must resolve. There are a number of other questions which must be addressed prior to the primary data collection actually being performed. How these questions are answered may serve to limit or modify the assessment techniques employed and/or necessitate the collection of additional data, as well as provide a framework for the interpretation of findings yielded by the assessment. In this paper we shall focus on several broad overlapping sets of concerns which demand attention in almost all procedures for assessing the need for preventive services for children. These include: (1) the parameters of the population that programs are to be targeted toward, (2) the resources which are already available and "in place" with objectives similar to that of the proposed program, and (3) the assessment of utilization. All of these concerns, as they relate to non-primary prevention programs, have been discussed elsewhere to varying degrees (e.g., Kamis, 1979; Zautra & Simons, 1978). For prevention planning, however, there are important differences in the nature of the issues involved that can lead to problems for those who are accustomed to thinking in terms of more traditional services.

The question of what parameters to use to determine the target population for preventive services is much more ambiguous, at least on some levels, than in the case of traditional clinical services. In the latter case, the target population is clear, concern is with those children who are already displaying emotional dysfunction. By contrast, ideally the goal for mental health agencies concerned with prevention is to develop and implement prevention programming for all "other," i.e., "healthy," children. If this were possible, the question of target population for preventive services would be simple. Unfortunately, human and financial resource limitations inevitably lead to the necessity of assigning higher programming priorities to some subgroups of this large "healthy" population over others. Appropriately, the question may be raised as to whether this is not in fact why we do a needs assessment. It should be recognized, however, that the same resource limitations which constrain the level of programming offered also constrain the scope of the needs assessment procedures which can be executed successfully. Consequently, before a formal collection of needs data is accomplished some decisions about the targeting of the needs assessment must be made.

No clear rules exist to aid in deciding what groups of children should be the focus of efforts to assess the need for preventive services. Assuredly, however, it is not an effective expenditure of resources to engage in assessment activities which identify needs for which viable programs cannot be developed. Thus, prior to designing an assessment strategy it is important to have a clear understanding and "pre-assessment" of those factors which may bear on the nature of programs which can be successfully implemented. Such factors include knowledge of the skills and orientations of the individuals in the agency developing the program, the availability of external resources, including cooperating agencies and settings, and public attitudes toward various forms of preventive efforts. For example, we may preliminarily decide to develop an assessment plan to identify the need for social competence or enhancement programs targeted to all "healthy" children in a given area. Actually doing such an assessment, however, is of relatively little value unless there are individuals available who can implement it, cooperation from such key potential delivery settings as schools is available, and the community is in favor of it. In brief then, one key element which may be used to guide the targeting of effective formal assessments of need for preventive children's services is an informal assessment of the program implementation resources which are available.

A second key step in the needs assessment process is a careful determination of what services currently are available for the population of concern. Such information may be invaluable for determining subgroups of the healthy population of children for whom there are gaps in services. That is, while needs assessment techniques, particularly objective ones, may provide some indication of absolute need or level of risk present, they do not yield information on the extent to which these needs are currently being met (Gully, 1980). For example, the data yielded by a social indicators analysis may show one subgroup to be at greater risk than a second due to the presence of a higher level of environmental stress. It will not, however, reveal that the former group may have available to it a far greater array of existing support programs designed to enhance coping efforts than the latter group.

In the identification of existing programming there is a key point for mental health professionals to keep in mind when dealing with prevention efforts for children. That is, children toward whom prevention efforts are targeted are typically not those to whom mental health professionals are seen as having a primary or even a legitimate claim. Efforts deemed as preventive by mental health professionals may exist in other contexts and on other agencies' "turfs." For example, social competence building procedures may already be incorporated into the daily school routine or as part of Head Start. Mental health planners must be careful to attend to the involvements of settings and agencies not typically thought of as in the business of mental health in prevention related activities if they are to develop an accurate understanding of children's needs for services.

A third issue of importance in planning and evaluating assessments of need for preventive services for children is that of utilization. Potentially this is a much more knotty problem for prevention planners than for planners of more traditional mental health services. In the case of primary prevention services, the notion of demand for service may be difficult to apply. At the very least, a shift in our understanding of what constitutes service utilization is necessary to more closely match the goals and strategies of prevention.

There are a number of reasons for these differences which may be summarized briefly, although not exhaustively, into three sets of issues. First, rather than being passive-receptive in their orientation, as are more traditional services, prevention programs attempt to actively seek to bring their services to targeted individuals. Second, prevention programs are generally intended to serve groups before there is perceived need for such service at the individual level although, in the case of prevention efforts during major life events, this may be less true (Felner, Norton, Cowen, & Farber, 1981) then when dealing with programming such as that aimed at competence enhancement or affective education. Third, while in some instances it is possible to count individuals served by prevention programs, much as we can "cases" in traditional services, in other instances this may not be possible. Cowen (1980) has pointed out that prevention programs can be directly targeted, where the benefits are for the actual participants, or indirectly targeted, where individuals have significant shaping interaction with the ultimate target groups. Directly targeted programs might include crisis intervention efforts or the development of social support groups while indirectly targeted efforts may include consultation or mental health education. In the case of the former programs, it may be possible to assess actual numbers of individuals utilizing the program. However, clearly, in the case of indirectly targeted services, it is often exceedingly difficult or impossible to assess the number of actual recipients of program benefits.

Utilization rates, then, may not provide an accurate or even appropriate benchmark against which to evaluate prevention needs assessment efforts or programs. Even when utilization rate can be determined, it should be clear from the foregoing that the rate of "client" use may be less a function of actual demand for services, in the traditional sense, than of the efficacy of the program's efforts to reach its target group.

In summary, in assessing the need for preventive services for children, it is important to understand the ways the differences in the goals and objectives of prevention, as opposed to those underlying more traditional mental health services, serve to change the issues which must be considered in planning and evaluating such procedures. Conceptions of what constitutes a need, strategies for identifying target groups, and approaches to evaluating demand for and/or utilization of service are but a few of the issues involved in planning for preventive children's services which require a clear understanding of differences between preventive and reconstructive mental health paradigms if they are to be adequately resolved.

REFERENCES

Baker, M. (Ed.). *The design of human service systems.* Wellesley, Mass.: The Human Ecology Institute, 1974.

Birtchnell, J. The possible consequences of early parent death. *British Journal of Medical Psychiatry,* 1964, *42,* 1-12.

Bloom, B.L. Prevention of mental disorders: Recent advances in theory and practice. *Community Mental Health Journal,* 1979, *15,* 179-191.

Cochran, N. On the limiting properties of social indicators. *Evaluation and Program Planning,* 1974, *2,* 1-4.

Cowen, E.L. The wooing of primary prevention. *American Journal of Community Psychology,* 1980, *8,* 253-285.

Cowen, E.L. Primary prevention in mental health: Past, present, and future. In R.D. Felner, L.A. Jason, J. Moritsugu, & S.S. Farber (Eds.), *Preventive psychology: Theory, research, and practice.* New York: Pergamon Press, 1983.

Cox, G.B., Carmichael, S.J., & Dightman, C.R. The optional treatment approach to needs assessment. *Evaluation and Program Planning,* 1979, *2,* 269-275.

Dohrenwend, B. Social stress and community psychology. *American Journal of Community Psychology,* 1978, *6,* 1-14.

Felner, R.D., Farber, S.S., and Primavera, J. Children of divorce, stressful life events, and transitions: A framework for preventive efforts. In R.H. Price, R.K. Ketterer, B.C. Bader, & J. Monahan (Eds.), *Prevention in mental health: Research, policy, and practice.* Beverly Hills: Sage, 1980.

Felner, R.D., Ginter, M.A., Boike, M.F., & Cowen, E.L. Parental death or divorce and the school adjustment of young children. *American Journal of Community Psychology,* 1981, *9,* 181-191.

Felner, R.D., Norton, P., Cowen, E.L., & Farber, S.S. A prevention program for children experiencing life crises. *Professional Psychology,* 1981, *12,* 446-452.

Felner, R.D., Primavera, J., & Cauce, A.M. The impact of school transitions: A focus for preventive efforts. *American Journal of Community Psychology,* 1981, *9,* 449-459.

Gersten, J.C., Langner, T.S., Eisenberg, J.G., & Simcha-Fagen, O. An evaluation of the etiologic role of stressful life-change events in psychological disorders. *Journal of Health and Social Behavior,* 1977, *18,* 228-244.

Jessner, L., Blom, G.E., & Waldfogel, S. Emotional implications of tonsilectomy and adnoidectomy in children. In R.D. Eisslen (Ed.), *The psychoanalytic study of the child.* New York: International Universities Press, 1952.

Kamis, E. A witness for the defense of need assessment. *Evaluation and Program Planning,* 1979, *2,* 7-12.

Legg, C., Sherick, I., & Wadland, W. Reactions of preschool children to the birth of a sibling. *Child Psychiatry and Human Development,* 1974, *5,* 3-39.

Nguyen, T.D., Attkisson, C.C., & Bottino, M.J. *Definition and identification of human service need in a community context.* Paper presented at the Conference on Needs Assessment in Health and Human Services, Louisville, Kentucky, 1976.

Padilla, E.R., Padilla, A.M., Morales, A., Olmedo, E.L., & Ramirez, R. Inhalant, marijuana and alcohol abuse among barrio children and adolescents. *International Journal of the Addictions,* 1979, *14,* 943-964.

Price, R.H., Bader, B.C., & Ketterer, R.F. Prevention in community mental health: The state of the art. In R.H. Price, R.F. Ketterer, B.C. Bader, & J. Monahan (Eds.), *Prevention in mental health: Research, policy, and practice.* Beverly Hills: Sage, 1980.

Report to the President from the President's Commission on Mental Health. Washington, D.C.: U.S. Government Printing Office, 1978.

Warheit, G.J., Buhl, J.M., & Bell, R.A. A critique of social indicators analysis and key informants surveys as needs assessment methods. *Evaluation and Program Planning,* 1978, *1,* 239-247.

Zautra, A., & Simons, L.S. An assessment of a community's mental health needs. *American Journal of Community Psychology,* 1978, *6,* 351-362.

A Needs Assessment
of Human Service Agencies
in an Urban Community

Gregory J. Meissen
Joseph A. Cipriani

ABSTRACT. Research and interventions aimed at maximizing the impact and organizational effectiveness of human service agencies, as well as the system of agencies in a community, could have far reaching effects on the large number of individuals served by these agencies. But prior to any type of active intervention it is imperative to document the needs and resources of these agencies. The present study was conducted to better understand (1) the functioning of individual agencies, (2) their role in the human service community, (3) the general workings of the urban human service community prior to any type of intervention, and (4) to provide a baseline to monitor changes in the human service community. Ninety-two non-profit human service agencies were surveyed in an urban setting. The results indicated that agency administrators were deeply concerned about funding problems, issues of accountability, and personnel concerns while reporting staff expertise, public relations, and efficient use of resources as agency strengths. Suggestions for interventions centered on using various agency strengths, as well as other community experts, to assist human service agencies. Special areas of concern were preventing the discontinuation of services through agency closings and developing a "networking" approach to help agencies adapt to recent changes in social policy.

Human services offered in our society are presently undergoing a dramatic change. The implications of extensive cuts in federal support to social services are difficult to predict, but it is evident that the structure and level of human service organizations will undergo a transition in the 80s. Research and interventions aimed at max-

This study was supported by Research and Sponsored Programs Grant # 3744-22, Wichita State University. All correspondence should be sent to Gregory J. Meissen, Department of Psychology, Wichita State University, Wichita, Kansas 67208.

123

imizing the impact and organizational effectiveness of human service agencies, as well as the system of agencies in a community, in order to prevent diminished services and agency closings could have far reaching effects on the large number of individuals served by these agencies. Cook and Campbell (1977) have suggested that a "call for change" without specific recommendations for action provides more flexibility for the applied researcher. But prior to any type of active intervention it is imperative to document the needs and resources of agencies as they enter this new era in social policy (Fairweather & Tornatzky, 1977; Murrell, 1973). Needs assessment techniques appear to be an appropriate method of obtaining this type of information.

A majority of needs assessment research has been directed at the individual level in order to estimate the extent of a disease or problem in a target population (Warheit, Bell, & Schwab, 1974). While this approach has proven to be useful, it rarely gives an indication of concomitant individual or community resources that could be used to mitigate the problem. Rarely has relevant information been obtained about both needs and resources to guide later interventions at the levels of human service organizations and the system in which they are embedded. Goodstein (1978) has encouraged organizational and systems level consultation as a more cost effective means of precipitating meaningful change for the individuals served by these organizations. In the past, attempts to alleviate pervasive problems that have been identified through needs assessment research have typically come in the form of new human service programs or changes in social policy prescribed for the afflicted population, a strategy not likely to prevail in the 80s. Further, most needs assessments using the individual as the unit of analysis have been limited to a specific problem (e.g., suicide, alcoholism) or, at best, have targeted one general type of problem (mental illness, physical health). A more rational strategy for improving the plight of troubled individuals would be to concentrate on maximizing the effectiveness of existing human service organizations and the community of services in general, so as to prevent the loss of these services during this critical time. This approach automatically considers the broad range of human concerns as "it is to such systems that troubled persons of all sorts turn for help—the emotionally disturbed, the retarded, the handicapped, and the impoverished" (Goodstein, 1978, p. 6).

A majority of organizational consultation, intervention and

research does not occur in non-profit human service agencies (Golembiewski, 1969). The activity that does take place is typically done on an agency by agency basis with little recognition of the larger aggregate of human services (e.g., Cherniss & Egnatios, 1978; Wilder & Gadlin, 1977). An alternative approach would be to routinely assess the organizational needs and resources of the human service community prior to these singular interventions. Therefore, the present study took the unusual approach of assessing the needs of human service organizations specifically in regard to improving the functioning and meeting the goals of the individual agencies. There was a special interest in the non-profit human service agencies as they face the new policies of the Reagan Administration. The study was also conducted to better understand (1) the functioning of the individual agencies, (2) their role in the human service community, (3) the general workings of the urban human service community prior to any type of intervention, and (4) to provide a baseline to monitor changes in the human service community.

METHOD

Sample

The original population consisted of 135 human service organizations from the metropolitan area of Wichita, Kansas. An organization needed to exhibit the following criteria in order to be included in this original population: (a) the primary activity of the agency was aimed at a human concern or a social service, and (b) the agency maintained a non-profit status. The primary sources used in identifying these agencies were the United Way Community Service Directory (1980), local telephone directories, and individuals knowledgeable about local human services. These individuals received preliminary lists of agencies for notable omissions and inappropriate inclusions. Larger human service institutions, such as hospitals, police departments, and school systems, were not included in the present study. Approximately 20 of the agencies from this original population were no longer in operation at the time of the interviews, which began approximately 60 days after the initial list of 135 agencies was constructed. From this final sampling frame of 115 agencies, 92 interviews were conducted. Personnel from five agencies refused interviews, and interviews could not be arranged at

17 agencies (e.g., respondents were on vacation or unable to schedule an appointment). Seventy interviews were conducted by paid interviewers at $6.00 per interview while the remaining 22 interviews were conducted by the investigators and graduate assistants.

Procedure

Interviewers were trained in basic interviewing techniques and were made familiar with the rationale of the project. After having an opportunity to familiarize themselves with the interview form, each interviewer conducted a "mock" interview with one of the investigators. Interviewers were then provided with the names, addresses, and telephone numbers of the agencies to be interviewed, as well as a person to contact at the target agency. All interviews were with an administrator in the target agency, with a majority (80%) being conducted with the executive director. The executive director, used as a key informant, was considered the one most appropriate individual to interview in the agency because of the diversity of information needed. Further, a majority of the questions were of an organizational, administrative or planning nature. While this approach was the most efficient, staff and client perceptions of the agency would have provided complimentary information if time had permitted. Interviews took place at the agency and lasted an average of 45 minutes. All interviews were completed between June 1 and June 26, 1981.

Interview Instrument

The instrument was a structured interview/questionnaire that consisted of six major sections including agency needs and strengths, staff characteristics, client characteristics, agency board characteristics, agency structure, and interorganizational characteristics. The section of the instrument from which a majority of information was taken for the present study was the agency needs and strengths section. This section focused on respondents' perceptions of: (a) agency strengths and resources, (b) areas where the strengths and expertise of the staff could be helpful to other, similar agencies, (c) agency needs and problems, and (d) areas where assistance from outside the agency would be particularly useful. Items targeting needs and strengths focused on the organizational functioning of the agency (e.g., funding concerns, staff and client concerns, accountability, agency structure). These items used a five point Likert-type scale on which respondents rated the perceived likelihood of assistance being needed in that particular area (1 = very likely; 2 = likely; 3 = perhaps; 4 = not likely; 5 = very unlikely). Respondents were also asked to prioritize, using an open ended format, the five most crucial agency needs/problems, the five problem areas in most need of outside assistance, where they would obtain such assistance, and the five areas of the agency considered to be the strongest or where staff could most productively consult with other agencies.

RESULTS AND DISCUSSION

Overview of Human Service Community

The size of the organizations, as measured by total number of employees, ranged from one employee to a total of 214 staff. The average staff size was 22 employees. The total number of employees for all human service agencies interviewed was 2071, with 1270 or 61% of the staff in positions with direct client contact, another 379 or 18% primarily concerned with administrative duties, and the remaining 422 or 21% in clerical, maintenance, and other types of positions. Of the 2071 employees, 409 or 20% held a masters degree or better, 666 or 32% had bachelors level training, and 996 or 48% had less than a bachelors degree. Of the 92 agencies in the sample 65% had paraprofessionals involved in the agency, with all but five agencies allowing them direct client contact. Further, 87% reported they were either satisfied or very satisfied with the performance of these paraprofessionals.

The characteristics of clients in this human service community were as varied as Goodstein (1978) assumed. Approximately 69 different types of clients were served by the 92 agencies, ranging from disaster victims to abused children to displaced homemakers. These clients were primarily white (72%), with blacks making up 18% of the client population (the population of Wichita is about 15% black). The remaining 10% of clients were Hispanic (4%), Native American (4%), or Oriental (2%). The agencies, in general, served slightly more females (55%) than males. Ages of clients ranged from a few days after birth to well into the 90s.

The most frequent type of service offered across all the agencies was counseling which included individual, group and family counseling. About 36% considered this type of service a major function of the agency. A relatively large percentage of agencies (34%) reported that health related concerns were a major focus of service provision. Another service often mentioned was public education, with 29% of the agencies reporting this to be a primary service objective. Approximately 23% of the agencies specifically mentioned that referral of clients was a routine service provided. Other frequently mentioned areas included services for youth (18%), drug/alcohol programs (14%), handicapped services (9%), and concerns of the elderly (8%).

Needs and Strengths

The results indicated that respondents were deeply concerned with funding problems as their organizations entered the 1980s. Eighty percent listed funding problems as one of the five most crucial needs of the agency with 68% of those agencies considering funding problems as their first priority. When asked specific questions regarding funding issues, 55.4% of the respondents indicated a need for outside assistance with fund raising in general. About 58% showed an interest in developing corporate funding sources and identifying new sources of funding with some outside assistance. About 47% reported a need for assistance in grant writing and obtaining federal grants.

Though it is apparent that funding is a serious concern at this time, funding problems always have and always will be a most serious issue as they are so closely tied to "organizational survival" (Katz & Kahn, 1978). Without prior longitudinal data, it was difficult to assess the impact of recent budgetary and policy changes, but a number of respondents expressed an increasingly greater concern about the "funding situation." More than a few predicted the close of their agency prior to the beginning of the next fiscal year. Historically, social scientists have avoided funding concerns because of a lack of expertise in that area. Unfortunately, most agencies did not report an expertise in fund raising either. Only 4% of respondents indicated that fund raising activities were an agency strength. The continuation of this avoidance of funding concerns can have increasingly greater consequences, with a major repercussion being the loss of services of those agencies most "at risk." The "at risk" agency is typically the small or new agency, and/or the agency dealing with minority populations or sensitive social issues.

A number of respondents expressed a need for improvement in the area labeled accountability (see Table 1). While only 17.4% indicated a need for assistance in the decision making process, 37% thought it likely or very likely they needed assistance in the analysis of agency data to be used in making decisions or supporting accreditations. About 42% saw a need to obtain help in improving or developing a management information system to routinely assist administrators in day to day decision making. Program evaluation and needs assessments were also seen by about 45% of the respondents

Table 1

Perceived Likelihood of Assistance Needed

Perceived Need For Assistance	Likely or Very Likely	Unlikely or Very Unlikely
Accountability		
Agency Decision Process	17.4%	52.2%*
Management Info System	42.4%	52.2%
Data analysis for Decisions	37.0%	32.6%
Data analysis Accreditations	37.0%	40.2%
Program Evaluation	45.7%	28.3%
Needs Assessment	44.6%	20.7%
Research Activities	37.0%	33.7%
Funding Concerns		
Fund Raising	55.4%	22.9%
Obtaining Federal Grants	46.7%	41.3%
Identifying New Funding	57.6%	16.3%
Corporate Funding	57.6%	25.0%
Grant Writing	46.7%	38.0%
Personnel Concerns		
Staff Recruitment	42.4%	34.7%
Staff Training/Orientation	41.3%	37.0%
Staff Turnover	23.9%	56.5%
Staff Absenteeism	7.6%	78.2%
Staff Burnout	37.0%	33.7%
Client Concerns		
Greater Number of Clients	34.8%	23.9%
More Appropriate Clients	22.8%	60.9%
Client Screening	20.7%	66.3%
Client Follow-up	34.8%	39.1%
Agency Structure		
Development Agency Goals	27.2%	52.2%
Development Agency Structure	18.5%	51.1%
Reorganization of Board	19.6%	58.7%
Recruitment of Board Members	39.1%	39.1%

N = 92
* Percentages do not equal 100 due to elimination of the neutral response of "perhaps" which indicated uncertainty concerning perceived need for assistance.

as being areas where outside assistance would be useful, even though 61% of the agencies attempted to evaluate the effectiveness of their services and 50% performed assessments of the level of need in the community for their services. It appeared that most of this activity was precipitated by accreditation procedures or grant requirements, as 70% of the agencies were routinely monitored by at least one regulatory group for various reasons (e.g., certifications, accreditations, legislative review, audits). A related finding was that 37% thought it likely to very likely that a need existed for research expertise in the agency, as opposed to about 34% who thought this need unlikely or very unlikely.

Another area which showed a relatively high level of need was personnel concerns (see Table 1). Though 71% of the agencies had training/orientation procedures for new staff members, 42% of the respondents indicated a need for outside assistance in this area. Also, about 42% of the respondents expressed a need for better staff recruitment procedures. Further, only 10% indicated that it was easy or very easy to hire qualified staff. A related concern was "staff burnout," with 37% of the respondents indicating an interest in outside assistance in this area. It appears that it is difficult to hire, train or retain quality staff in these human service organizations. These findings are not inconsistent with prior research on personnel problems in human services and specifically in the area of staff burnout (e.g., Abels, 1977; Cherniss, 1980a; Cherniss, 1980b).

When respondents were asked to list the five areas where the agency was strongest or had a great amount of resources, a broad range of strengths was reported. Of the 85 different strengths elicited, staff expertise was the most frequently mentioned with 36% of the respondents considering it an important resource. A typical comment regarding staff expertise was "our staff seem unusually capable in tough counseling situations. Other frequently mentioned strengths were good public relations in the community (25%) and with other agencies (14%), efficient services and use of agency resources (20%), and an ability to recruit and train volunteers (15%). At the same time, lack of qualified staff was considered a problem in 36% of the agencies, public relations a deficit in 29%, and lack of volunteers a problem in 19% of the agencies in this sample. It is apparent that the strengths and resources of some agencies were considered a most crucial problem in others. If agency staff and administrators who have expertise in areas such as public relations and volunteer recruitment could share relevant information with agencies deficient in these areas, those individuals served by the human service community could profit (Sarason, Carroll, Maton, Cohen, & Lorentz, 1977; Sarason & Lorentz, 1979).

Implications for Action

The results of the present study provide a useful framework for the proposal of specific interventions in the community of human services. Many of these interventions center on the concept of "networking" among individual human service agencies with the goal being more efficient and effective agencies without a large increase of resources. One can conceptualize many of these interventions as being of a preventative nature with the organization as the unit of analysis. These interventions are structured around maximizing resources during a period of social policy emphasizing severe cutbacks, reduction of client services, and agency closings. Such interventions can lead to the development of a more viable "network" of human service agencies, and prevent the demise of agencies which can make a contribution to this network. This type of networking and prevention activity could be based in the consultation and education unit of a community mental health center or be sponsored by the United Way.

An intervention that could have effects on a major portion of a human service community is a cooperative exchange of agency expertise. The results of the present study indicate that what are strengths for some agencies are problems for others. The concept of a "system of exchange" could be instituted, with a broker matching existing strengths with requests for assistance, and monitoring the contributions and receiving of assistance by individual agencies. Individual agencies could enhance their organizational efficiency by paying with their own expertise instead of money.

A related proposal would establish a central consultation service for non-profit organizations. In order to be cost-effective, such a service would need to be staffed primarily by volunteer experts (e.g., retired businesspersons and agency personnel, university staff and students, agency administrators), who could contribute a few hours of their expertise per year to non-profit agencies in the community. These groups of experienced individuals could assist human service organizations on a variety of important concerns, such as fund raising and agency board development.

Agency board development is a specific intervention with potential for extensive improvement in the functioning of a human service community. About 20% of the respondents of this study indicated that they were likely or very likely to need assistance in board reorganization, and about 39% reported assistance was desired in the recruitment of new board members (see Table 1). Agency boards are often amenable to reorganization because of the considerable change of membership on a yearly basis. Systematic efforts made to educate agency administrators and board members on how to create a board, how to analyze agency needs for specific types of board members, how to recruit desirable members, and how to maximize their impact on the agency can clearly have a positive effect on the organization. A well functioning board of directors or client advisory board can assist agency personnel in many of the operations that insure a viable service to consumers (Zald, 1974; Silverman, 1981).

In the area of accountability and planning, annual or semi-annual assessments of the needs and strengths of these non-profit agencies could complement regular surveys of citizen needs concerning human services. Murrell and Schulte (1980) have conducted tri-annual surveys for the last four years in order to "take the pulse" of the community and to be a source of objective information for community decision makers, agencies and citizen groups. Routine area-wide needs assessments of agencies and citizen surveys would not only provide relevant data for rational decision making, but would also be the basis for longitudinal research on interventions and local policy changes.

CONCLUSIONS

The unusual approach of assessing the needs of an urban human service community provided preliminary data that can guide future research and interventions in human service systems. Information was collected with a focus on the needs and strengths of agencies, as perceived by agency administrators, as they entered this new era of social policy. The implications of the study were not oriented towards monetary solutions, but encouraged the development of more cost-efficient interventions to allow agencies to help themselves and each other. Through needs assessments and survey research, social scientists have the skills and methods to provide objective information, which can be an invaluable framework for empirically based decision-making and intervention in human service systems.

REFERENCES

Abels, P. *The new practice of supervision and staff development.* New York: Association Press, 1977.
Cherniss, C., & Egnatios, E. Is there job satisfaction in community mental health? *Community Mental Health Journal,* 1978, *14,* 309-318.
Cherniss, C. *Professional burnout in human services organizations.* New York: Praeger, 1980a.
Cherniss, C. Organizational design and human service programs. In R.H. Price & P.E. Politser (Eds.), *Evaluation and action in the social environment.* New York: Academic Press, 1980b.
Cook, T.D., & Campbell, D.T. The design and conduct of quasi-experiments and true experiments in field settings. In I.M. Dunnette (Ed.), *Handbook of industrial/organizational psychology.* New York: Rand McNally, 1976.
Fairweather, G.W., & Tornatzky, L.G. *Experimental methods for social policy research.* Elmsford, New York: Pergamon Press, 1977.
Golembiewski, R.T. Organizational development in public agencies: Perspectives on theory and practice. *Public Administration Review,* 1969, *29,* 367-378.
Goodstein, L.D. *Consulting with human service systems.* Reading, Mass.: Addison-Wesley, 1978.
Katz, D., & Kahn, R.L. *The social psychology of organizations.* New York: John Wiley & Sons, 1978.
Murrell, S.A. *Community psychology and social systems: A conceptual framework and intervention guide.* New York: Behavioral Publications, 1973.
Murrell, S.A., & Schulte, P. A procedure for systematic citizen input to community decision-making, *American Journal of Community Psychology,* 1980, *8,* 19-30.
Sarason, S.B., Carroll, C.F., Maton, K., Cohen, S., & Lorentz, E. *Human services and resource networks.* San Francisco: Jossey-Bass, 1977.
Sarason, S.B., & Lorentz, E. *The challenge of the resource exchange network.* San Francisco: Jossey-Bass, 1979.
Silverman, W.H. Self-designed training for mental health advisory/governing boards. *American Journal of Community Psychology,* 1981, *9,* 67-82.
United Way Community Service Directory of Wichita and Sedgwick County. Wichita, KS: United Way of Wichita and Sedgwick County, 1980.
Warheit, G.J., Bell, R.A., & Schwab, J.J. *Planning for change: Needs assessment approaches.* Washington, D.C.: National Institute of Mental Health, 1974.
Wilder, J.F., & Gadlin, W. A halfway house in mental health center. *Community Mental Health Journal,* 1977, *13,* 168-174.
Zald, M.N. The power and functions of board of directors: A theoretical synthesis. In Y. Hasenfeld & R.A. English (Eds.), *Human service organizations.* Ann Arbor: University of Michigan Press, 1974.